VITAMIN C
THE PROS AND CONS

Stephen Sheffrey, D.D.S.

Prion Books

Copyright © 1991 by Stephen Sheffrey
All rights reserved
ISBN: 0-9629372-0-7

Library of Congress   91-90308

Prion Books
P.O. Box 8194
Ann Arbor, Michigan 48107

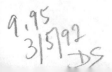

To the memory of Tom

Contents

1
The Depleters

Whatever you want to call it—vitamin C, ascorbic acid, ascorbate or just C—this unique substance acts as a vitamin in low doses, as a drug in high doses and as a general handyman at dose levels in between. Its versatility accounts for the intense interest which generates about 300 published professional items worldwide every year relating to its medical properties—more than one every working day.

The basic function of C is of course as a vitamin necessary for the prevention of scurvy. Most individuals can be protected from this condition by a daily intake of about 10 milligrams. The optimal body reserve can be maintained in many of us when our food or a pill supplies the recommended daily allowance (RDA) of 60 milligrams. That amount keeps our blood plasma level in the normal range of .4 to 1.1 milligrams of C per deciliter. Some tables list the high normal at 1.5 milligrams per deciliter. A deciliter is a little less than a half cup.

The high normal of 1.5 milligrams per deciliter is roughly the "saturation point" or "renal threshold."

Urinary excretion of C rises substantially when an extra amount is taken while its plasma level is at the saturation point. This has led to the belief by some authorities that taking more than a gram a day is useless because much of it is eliminated within 4 hours via the urine. When the body is sick the normal urinary excretion of C may drop to zero because the body needs more when sick. The daily urinary excretion of C during health depends on intake and individual differences. About 40 milligrams, plus or minus 30 is the normal range.

Except for the guinea pig, a couple of bat species and the primates, including humans, all mammal species can make their own C internally. It is interesting to note that their plasma C level is normally maintained at or near the saturation point. When such an animal is stressed it produces more C for the body to utilize. The rat, for example, will increase production several fold (from G. Dettman's reproduction of Irwin Stone's table, 1976). Humans cannot do this. Extra C must be taken orally or injected.

Any stress or trauma, whether physical or mental, depletes the human body of C. *There are other depleters also. We should become aware of them.* Even without considering depleters, too many of us are down substantially in our blood level of the vitamin, as several authorities have stated. We may be getting along okay but we are not at our best and there's no reserve if we should need it. G. Goldsmith in 1961 and C.W.M. Wilson in 1974 stated that humans might fare better if their plasma C levels were maintained at the saturation point where C-making species keep it.

Just because the diet supplies the recommended daily allowance doesn't mean that it is enough in all instances. Some authorities believe the RDA is too low regardless. Soviet citizens fare better in this area. The recommended daily intake over there is 125 milligrams, more than twice what we are advised to take. Even that amount will not satisfy the requirement of everyone because the way we live is a factor in how much we need.

And, as different individuals, we use C at different rates. The sailors who developed scurvy on those long voyages didn't all become sick on the same day. A few even managed to stay healthy. When Jacques Cartier's 110 men wintered on an island in the St. Lawrence in 1535–36, 3 or 4 of them were still functioning normally at the spring thaw in the middle of April. But 25 had died, the condition of 40 others appeared hopeless and the rest were down with varying degrees of scurvy. At that point they learned of an Indian brew made from the bark and leaves of an evergreen. They stripped a huge tree and cured themselves in 8 days. Afterward, it is said, the evergreen was named arborvitae—tree of life.

Those few who didn't get scurvy must have been able to keep going on very little C. Or they had access to food containing it or they could make it internally as most mammal species do. Nobody has ever found a human who could make C internally but the thought surfaces occasionally. The fact that captains have come through the long voyages better than their crews suggests that captains and the few who could sneak a bite of his better cuisine were getting more C. Historical accounts don't tell much about the duties of the survivors.

But all survivors couldn't have dipped a finger into the captain's food supply. Some bodies are simply more efficient in the use of C. This was shown by R.E. Hodges in 1969 and 1971 with studies on a total of 9 men given a diet devoid of C so that they had to draw on their body reserve. One man's metabolism used 2.2 percent of his C reserve each day while another squandered 4.1 percent. If a man who used almost twice the C as another could be found in a group of 9, how great a difference would we find in a thousand, or a million? Nobody knows what the extremes are.

VanderKamp (1966) used a color-change reaction to determine the amount of C the body could use before a certain portion of it appeared in the urine to change the color of a testing liquid. He saw the color change after healthy individuals took an average of 4 grams a day. But 40 grams a day, on average, were taken before that same color change occurred when schizophrenics took the test. This suggests that they need 10 times more C than others. Indeed, for years Abram Hoffer treated schizophrenics with high doses of C. He mentioned a case in 1967 of a patient being able to function again after taking a gram of C every hour for 2 days. The total dose was 45 grams, including make-up doses of a gram for each hour of sleep.

A 1986 paper by Suboticanec states that schizophrenics have lower plasma C levels than others and that populations with the highest rate of schizophrenia were lower in consumption of vitamin C. In 1987 Beauclair reported favorable results in 10 of 13 schizophrenics who took 8 grams of C daily. The treatment is not a cure but is helpful and is appreciated by the patients.

In the light of these findings one might think that every such patient would be given high C on a trial basis to check for improvement. Unfortunately, the vitamin is not a substance owned by a single company that can see a financial advantage in promoting it rather than a proprietary drug for the disease. Therefore not much attention is paid to these favorable reports. We'll see more examples of this in later chapters.

In addition to inborn differences in rates of use, certain habits, lifestyles and drugs draw down body stores of C. Two aspirin taken occasionally have little effect on the blood picture with respect to C but a couple of aspirin every 6 hours for a week will drop the amount of C carried by the white cells to half what it should be (Loh, 1973). The C that should stay in the body goes out in the urine.

This brings to mind the experience of Norman Cousins. He developed a type of arthritis diagnosed as ankylosing spondylitis. The chance of cure, his doctor said, was 1 in 500. In an article in the New England Journal of Medicine several years later (1976), Cousins recalled that he was taking 26 aspirin tablets a day along with other drugs. He was a very sick man.

One day a dormant instinct that stirred only after the outlook seemed hopeless thrust up a daring urge to change direction—or maybe he remembered that he'd read about high-C therapy. Whatever, he asked to be given 10 grams of C intravenously, plus more the next day and the next, up to 25 grams daily within a week. The doctor said such doses had never been given.

Now there is the sort of patient we may wish ourselves to be—bold enough to tell the doctor to try something. Cousins could do so because he was a biggie. And, as an editor he had access to ink by the barrel. The old saying that you can never win an argument against someone having those assets has never been proved scientifically. Nevertheless, the doctor didn't wait on science to refute it. He did as requested, not waiting on science to prove the value of C in such a case either.

Cousins improved quickly on the regimen and discontinued the pills. The book he wrote later mentions C briefly but most of the credit for recovery is given to laughter and the power of positive thinking. Such is the lot of vitamin C.

Whenever you've been put on tetracycline, the chances are that you have not been told to take extra C also. Shah reported in 1968 that the antibiotic dropped both the white-cell and plasma C. In 1972 Windsor wrote that a gram of tetracycline daily for 5 days lowered the white-cell C as much as several aspirins do. Although the dosing was stopped at day 5 the depletion continued until day 8. This of course lowers the ability of white cells to function at their peak so that the tetracycline is not as effective as it could be. Whether scurvy would occur after long-term heavy dosing is not known but a near-scurvy condition is bad enough, particularly when extra C is known to increase white-cell function and the effectiveness of some antibiotics (Rawal, 1974).

How many other drugs deplete the body of C is still a question. So many have not been investigated for this problem. Estrogen has, however. The Briggs couple reported in 1972 and '73 that estrogen and contraceptives containing it lower white-cell C levels significantly. They advised that extra C be taken to compensate.

About the white-cell C level: it is judged to be a more accurate gauge of body C stores than is the plasma level. The plasma level varies with the amount of C in the immediate diet while the white-cell (leukocyte) C reflects a longer-term dietary supply. Measuring it is more tedious, however, so that the plasma C in blood taken after a 6-hour fast is usually considered a fair gauge of how we're doing in the C department. *(But see page 146)*

A chemical in certain diet pills, fenfluramine, also lowers the level of C. In fact the chemical appears to be more effective as the C level drops, according to C.W.M. Wilson's human trials reported in 1974 and '75. Taking this drug does not appear to be an ideal way to slim down.

Smoking is a big C depleter, as several studies have shown. McCormick wrote in 1952 that each cigaret costs the body 25 milligrams. Pelletier in 1968 reported that smokers have less than half the plasma

C that nonsmokers have. That same year Brooks and Grimshaw reported that plasma C levels of heavy smokers are down in the range of a person 40 years older. In 1981 Kallner calculated that smokers need a C intake of 140 milligrams a day in order to counter this depletion effect. Perhaps the Surgeon General should have that message printed on the packs.

Age was mentioned above. For years it has been common knowledge among authorities that, on average, women have higher levels of plasma C than men and that the levels in both sexes decline as we grow older. In Brooks' and Grimshaw's 1968 paper it is seen that at age 20 the average woman's blood plasma contains about 1.1 milligrams of C per deciliter. A man's level averages about .3 milligrams less. In other words the female of the species is favored with about 37 percent more plasma C than men.

The rate of decline with age is equal in both sexes. At 65, women are down to about .75 milligrams per deciliter and men check in with .45. Projected further at the same rate, men would reach the scurvy range in their 80s. This is not so very far off the mark, according to Cheraskin's reproduction of a table by Basu and Schorah in *Vitamin C in Health and Disease* (1981, Croom Helm Ltd, London). Printed in the AMA Journal (1985; 254:2894), it shows that about half of the institutionalized elderly are in that range and 3 quarters to almost all of them have leukocyte C levels in the near-scurvy range. This does affect their health. Cheraskin and Ringsdorf reported an interesting observation in 1979 and '81: Certain changes in the electrocardiogram appear as we age.

These changes were seen to be more pronounced in persons taking less than 100 milligrams of C daily than in those taking more than 400 milligrams daily.

Perhaps the higher level of C in women has something to do with their greater longevity and their physical toughness when adversity strikes. It has been reported that during the Crusades, while men suffered from severe scurvy women living under the same conditions were giving birth to live babies— even though pregnancy further depletes the mother. Nature prepares the fetus for the shock of birth by loading it with an abundance of C, robbing the mother if necessary. Slobody in 1946 and Hamil in 1947 showed that the plasma C of a fetus can be twice that of the mother.

One wonders if the mood changes which some women suffer after giving birth are due in part to vitamin C depletion. Nobody has looked into this, apparently. I can find no report in the medical literature on the blood level of C in women who suffer from the blues after the blessed event. Yet papers mention that mental depression is a common occurrence in scurvy and the near-scurvy condition called subclinical scurvy.

The stress of pregnancy and giving birth—*every* stress, as was mentioned, whether caused by trauma, surgery, disease, emotional upset or life in the fast lane, lowers the leukocyte C level. At first the drop was thought to mean that the leukocytes were giving up their C to body tissues. This may happen to a certain extent but the real reason for the drop is that certain white cells which carry more C are diluted by millions of low-C white cells pouring into the bloodstream during stress, dropping the *average* C content of the white-cell component of the blood. It's like filling out a battalion whose elite members have rockets with recruits having BB guns.

However it is explained, the drop is important. For example, it can be prevented with high doses of C whenever a cold strikes, thereby preventing a cold. Also, a blood study of stroke victims found that the leukocyte and plasma C levels of those who died were lower than the levels of the survivors. The lowest level was seen in the patient who died first (Hume, 1982). Unless extra C is given the levels remain low for days.

B.D. Vallance followed 12 heart-attack patients for 8 weeks and reported some interesting observations (1978). Half the patients received no C other than what the diet provided. Plasma and leukocyte C levels dropped far below normal and were still low even at the end of the study 8 weeks later. In some cases the plasma C level was zero. The body tissues were taking up all of it.

The other 6 patients received a gram of C every 4 hours in their intravenous fluid for 48 hours. Their C levels rose quickly from the lows seen at the start. They were given 2 grams of C per day orally afterward, which maintained the levels at the high normal position. The author made no comment on whether the patients taking C were better off but did state that a low blood level of C is not a satisfactory situation in view of the tissue-repair needs during recovery.

Several reports have documented that hospital patients have low levels of C. T.S. Wilson in 1973 noted that the death rate of elderly patients after 4 weeks of hospitalization reached 47 percent when leukocyte C fell to half the normal level. The death rate was only 10 percent in those whose C was normal.

Perhaps one of the reasons hospitals don't pay much attention to our level of C is that opinions differ on whether it is important. Crandon expressed the opinion that the fall in C after surgery is a factor in complications (1961). But S. Vallance in 1985 held the view that the effect of C is minimal. Considering, however, that cancers are said to be more numerous in tissues that are low in C it seems prudent to maintain high C levels rather than ignore the evidence against a state of deficiency.

Hospitals should determine the C status of every patient who enters for treatment but they don't. Just this little item would have saved a woman the ordeal of 6 laparotomies in 38 months in repeated efforts to determine the cause of internal bleeding. The surgeons kept cutting her open to ladle out blood and search her innards for the reason without ever considering until the last cut that she might be low on C. The signs of scurvy such as bleeding gums and rough skin with coiled hairs and capillary breakdown had not appeared. But the amount of C in her was barely measurable (Cooke & Milligan, 1977).

If we can rate depleters by the amount needed to oppose them the viruses would head the list. As we will see, the cold viruses require a rise in dose of at least 5 grams daily, starting at the first sniffle, in order to be effective. Klenner, an experienced advocate of high-C therapy, used many times that amount when treating the more vicious viral diseases.

Cathcart, another advocate, has built on Klenner's findings and provided interested practitioners with valuable details on the use of C. His papers are published in *Medical Hypotheses,* a journal that does not carry advertising. No journal editor eager for advertising revenue would ever again be granted an account from the pharmaceutical companies if he or she dared to publish any of Cathcart's papers (1981, 1984, 1985, 1986, 1991).

His flexible dose schedule is based on the amount of C needed by the body from hour to hour as determined by the mood of the gut. For example, the gut may get rid of all the C over 10 grams a day taken by a healthy person but may absorb more than 100 grams a day when that person is ill with the flu. In other words, a person can take that much—a little at a time—in a day without getting the trots when a virus is attacking. I have treated myself with 84 grams—4 grams an hour for 21 hours—to stay ahead of flu symptoms until the threat subsided.

Oh my God! you're thinking, *I'd be camped in the bathroom if I took that much!*

You surely would if you took it improperly. Improperly means taking too much at a time instead of dividing the dose; or sluicing it down into an empty stomach; or loading up when you don't need so much; or taking a bunch of hard tablets that won't dissolve until too far down in the gut. For some, it may be improper to take the acid form when sodium ascorbate or calcium ascorbate agrees with them better. Like everything else, proper use comes with adequate directions plus experience. C should be taken *after* food. Yung reported in 1981 that taking C after eating slows its course through the gut, allowing 25 percent more to be absorbed. Taking smaller amounts every 15 minutes produces similar results but is not practical for some individuals.

Cathcart found that about 80 percent of his patients, when well, could take 10 to 15 grams of C a day, divided into 4 doses, without getting diarrhea. Much more can be taken during illness. The sicker the patient, the more the absorption. Diarrhea does not occur until the body has all it can use. By taking more and more at frequent intervals when sick, the human is doing what the C-making animals are programmed naturally to do—make more internally and pour it into the system.

In Cathcart's experience, viral pneumonia, mononucleosis and AIDS are the viral illnesses that allow the highest doses before the diarrhea point is reached. He gave an AIDS patient more than a half pound of C daily for 14 days. A 98-pound woman took a pound in 2 days to treat acute mononucleosis. She was nearly well afterward but continued taking 20 to 30 grams daily for about 2 months.

The most effective dose of C during illness is that which is just short of causing diarrhea. *Anything less is almost useless on acute symptoms.* This may be the reason why some individuals cannot see any benefit in taking it—they don't take enough. There are those, however, whose bowels will not tolerate the necessary dose. They must be given C by injection.

Because bowel looseness is the best indicator of the dose required, the regulation of it must be left to an informed patient. The patient should be aware of whether the symptoms are getting worse or easing off because the diarrhea point is a moving target. It "moves away" to allow a higher dose when one becomes sicker. During recovery the point moves closer, requiring a quick downward adjustment of the dose. One can enjoy a sporting time of it as the symptoms wax and wane in response to undershooting or overshooting the target. Who says there aren't any new challenges in this world?

Fortunately, marksmanship improves with experience. And the bowel looseness is a benign sort, not the liquid hellfire of some types. Better the trots than severe flu and the miserable aches. These can be avoided when C is taken properly. In a day the bowel usually signals that dose reduction can begin.

But not always. One winter my "flu" did not follow this pattern. The symptoms were still strong after the second day, prompting me to take an antibiotic, which was more effective. This led to the suspicion that the illness was not viral flu but an imitation caused by bacteria—probably *Hemophilus influenzae,* the organism first thought to be the flu bug. Although scientists learned later that it wasn't the usual cause, it still deserves the name given it. *Hemophilus* is a bacterial villain, not a virus. The confusion caused by bacterial flu and colds, which do not respond as readily to high C, is a major reason why its value in treatment is disputed.

Although not a depleter, the inability of the body to absorb C should be mentioned. Most of the C ingested is absorbed in the upper part of the small intestine but some goes into the bloodstream via the stomach wall. The absorption process is impaired if those areas are diseased or surgerized. Cohen and Duncan in 1967 reported that leukocyte C levels in duodenal-ulcer patients were less than half the normal amount. Five months after surgery the levels were still low and not expected to reach normal unless more C was taken. Others have reported similar lows after such surgery, including the gut bypasses done for those wanting to lose weight.

Low stomach acidity as well as other diseases in the area can lead to a lack of C. Esselen and Fuller in 1939 cited a case of scurvy mentioned in the Italian medical literature that didn't respond to extra C taken orally. It was thought that low stomach acidity allowed certain colon bacteria to become established higher up in the gut where they destroyed the vitamin before it could be absorbed. Taking plenty of C in the acid form could overwhelm the bacteria and allow for better absorption. Young and James in 1942 identified the bacteria that enjoyed feasting on C and suggested that lemon juice would inhibit them.

We've now seen how a person can be low in C while on a diet said to be adequate. He or she could be a low absorber, a high user or the victim of a depleter. Any one or combination of these conditions can depress the blood level of C down near the scurvy range but nobody would suspect it. Subclinical scurvy, as the near-scurvy condition is called, is seldom recognized. Only a blood test plus the realization that a low-normal range may be a sick range for some would alert healthcare personnel. Otherwise the link to scurvy would not be apparent. Whatever the complaint—skin rash or eye problems or swollen legs—could be called *target-organ scurvy* because the disease can attack where one is most susceptible.

Weariness, always seen in scurvy, appears to linger as well in the subclinical type. *Chronic Fatigue Syndrome* has been featured in popular magazines lately. Is it nothing more than subclinical scurvy? The victim usually recalls that fatigue began after flu-like symptoms. Flu is a major C depleter. Viruses can remain in the body for years, such as the chickenpox virus that reactivates to cause shingles. Those that are less dormant could be continuous depleters. A poorly functioning immune system accompanies the fatigue—another hint that low C may be a factor. Pondering all this, it seems imprudent not to suspect subclinical scurvy, particularly since depression often accompanies the fatigue syndrome.

D. Gold investigated a group of chronic-fatigue patients, comparing them with normal individuals. The two major differences were immune system changes and signs of depression (1990). The blood study in this investigation was extensive—except that no mention was made of the C content. Healthcare personnel seem to have developed a blind spot with respect to C. It is always assumed that everyone has enough of it.

A person may recover from the fatigue after several months. This is consistent with a slow rebuilding of the body reserves of C. Some, however, remain in the weary state for years. A lady with that experience told of the smorgasbord of symptoms that took their turns at making her life miserable. She ate ravenously but lost weight, suggesting a malabsorption problem which of course would lower the uptake of C. She developed gum trouble, suggesting the nearness of scurvy. She became weak, confused, muscle-sore, unable to work and depressed, all conditions seen as scurvy comes on. And she smoked, just one more depleter which would keep her C level down.

Several specialists could find nothing wrong with her. Only a little more iron in her system than normal. How interesting! *A direct result of excess iron in body tissues is a low blood level of C* (Lynch, 1967; Wapnick, 1969). Another depleter at work.

I mentioned the connection then asked if the C level of her blood had been checked. She said no. Having relatives in the healthcare system, she knew what tests had been done. I suggested that a gram of C after each meal would be an inexpensive way to diagnose subclinical scurvy because it would be curative unless other factors required taking even more C. But first she should have the iron removed. More on this problem later.

A month later I learned that she hadn't tried the regimen. Having relatives who were well indoctrinated in the ways of modern therapy—and afflicted with the usual blind spot—she was reluctant to try anything that lacked scientific proof of benefit for her specific disease. Whether she followed my last suggestion and had the C status of her body determined is not known.

Another "baffling medical problem" that becomes newsworthy from time to time is the reaction of a small percentage of women to a German measles vaccine. Women are advised to be vaccinated if they plan to have children because getting the virus during pregnancy can damage the fetus. The reaction the women suffer has some similarities to the fatigue syndrome. They're weak and weary and their lives are disrupted for months. The live virus used in the vaccine, although not infectious to anyone else, appears to linger in those few women at a subclinical stage that has its ups and downs.

Kalokerinos in 1976 criticized the vaccination of malnourished children as an "immunological insult" to their bodies. It is probably no less of an insult to the body of an adult who is low in C. I asked a physician who was treating a group of women having the post-vaccination reaction if he had determined the level of C in any of them. He said no. He didn't seem to feel that it was important. And, being unaware of the antiviral capability of C, he didn't realize that high doses could eliminate the lingering virus and restore the level of C in the process.

Individuals who regularly form calcium oxalate kidney stones are said to have low levels of C. More about this later. And anyone having intestinal parasites is a candidate for low C. In 1984 Cathcart advised clearing them out so that high C would be more effective in AIDS treatment. Some parasites manage to survive in the body by continuously shedding phony targets for the body's immune system to fight. It's a constant drain on the system and on C. Hawthorne and Storvick reported in 1948 that taking large amounts of sodium bicarbonate regularly drops the C level. The dose used was rather high, perhaps more than is generally used but is something to keep in mind. There may be other depleters that haven't been discovered yet or not mentioned because they're in the category of stress or malnutrition. The resilience of the human body is marvelous to behold in view of the C-grabbing possibilities that we live with.

2
Anatomy of a
Snow Job

One of the purposes of this book is to set the record straight, to point out the misconceptions about vitamin C that have accumulated over the years. One of these relates to whether it can ward off the common (viral) cold. Health columns and newsletters address this question perennially and consistently state that it cannot.

If you should ask a number of your friends about the assertion you're apt to collect three different answers, as I did: 1) "It doesn't help me. Nothing does." 2) "Maybe it's some good. I don't have as much misery when I take some." 3) "Hey, it's great stuff! I *never* get colds anymore!"

Those who make statement number three probably already know that scientific trials have not shown that vitamin C can prevent the common cold. How can they claim a benefit that science has found to be lacking? Let us examine the medical literature carefully to answer that question.

Medical experiments with vitamin C increased rapidly after its synthesis in the early 1930s. Its antiviral potential was of particular interest. Jungeblut, a New York scientist, reported in 1935 that he had inactivated the virus of poliomyelitis by injecting the vitamin into infected monkeys. Dainow, formerly of the dermatology clinic at the University of Geneva, reported case histories in 1936 then called vitamin C the medicine of choice for treating oral and genital herpes and shingles.

Pharmaceutical companies soon began promoting brand names of it to doctors. Merck's full-page ad in the *Journal of the American Medical Association* in 1937 recommended its brand only for scurvy and related conditions but the following year's ad (12–17–38) cited new research and expanded its use to infectious diseases and febrile conditions. The largest tablet contained 100 milligrams of C.

Physicians were not aware that the average adult in Ireland was getting 6 to 10 times that amount in the daily diet a century before. Rhoades wrote in the *National Geographic* in 1982 that each of those hard-working men and women consumed 9 to 14 pounds of potatoes a day. A pound of potatoes, boiled, contains 72 milligrams of C and provides about 318 calories. The diet supported a population density greater than that of modern-day China.

As one might expect, the vitamin was soon tried against the common cold. After a 2-year trial Ruskin reported in 1938 on 100 cold sufferers who had been injected with a calcium salt of vitamin C (calcium ascorbate). He saw marked improvement or complete relief in nearly all cases. But he attributed the benefit to the calcium.

Cowan's scientific trial reported in 1942 used oral doses up to a half gram daily—about as much as an underfed Irishman consumed long ago. Compared to a placebo, Cowan found that the small amount did provide a slight benefit. In 1947 the Australian physician Markwell reported good results with larger doses—three quarters of a gram or more as soon as a cold strikes plus a half gram or more every 3 or 4 hours afterward as needed. The "or more" could put the dose into double digits. The sooner the dose the better the response.

Cowan then tried higher doses, comparing C with and without antihistamines against a placebo (1950). He used two-thirds of a gram of C at the start plus the same amount every 4 hours. Participants in the trail were to continue dosing until symptoms vanished or the 10 tablets supplied were used up. Then they could request more if needed. If strictly followed, the intake would be 4 grams a day. Skipping the night dose would drop it to 3 and a third grams daily. The result: no significant benefit from all that C, whether taken alone or with antihistamines. Remember this trial. The results will be discussed later.

One man did like his "cold pills" enough to inquire later if they were on the market yet. On learning that they weren't, he made a long trip to pick up a supply from leftover stock. A look at the record then revealed that he had been in the group which took the placebo. Never underestimate the power of a placebo. Seven of those taking it reported reactions such as headache, nausea, swelling of the lip and increased frequency of urination. It is interesting that these reactions, except for the lip swelling, were also reported by the seven members of the C group who had reactions. None reported having bowel looseness.

After 5 years of experimenting the Massachusetts physician Regnier in 1968 put the minimum effective dose at 5 grams daily for 3 or 4 days. Dose timing is important, he stated. *The span between doses should not exceed 3 hours.* The amount of C that has left the bloodstream by then needs to be replenished. He advised 600 milligrams at the start of a cold, 750 at bedtime and also upon rising. The rest of the C should be divided into equal daytime doses to be taken not more than 3 hours apart.

An example: 600 milligrams is taken at the hint of a cold at 8 PM. At 11 PM bedtime 750 milligrams is taken, to be repeated after food in the morning. Assuming an 18-hour period before bedtime again, the 3½ grams allotted for this time is divided into 5 doses of 700 milligrams each and taken 3 hours apart. Or one could divide the daytime share into smaller doses to be taken more often.

The North Carolina physician Klenner reported on the treatment of viral diseases with high C in several papers published in the late forties and the fifties. For severe colds he advocated a gram an hour for 48 hours (1971). His philosophy of going beyond minimums reflects the reality that patients delay treatment, therefore need much larger doses plus antibiotics if bacterial invasion complicates the case.

His writings attest to long experience in the use of large amounts of C for treating all viral diseases, most notable a report of bringing 60 polio cases through an epidemic without the crippling that occurred in the area. One might think that the many accounts of successful treatments with C would encourage every doctor in the nation to use it. But other factors entered in. Vaccines and antibiotics were being developed, eliminating all the reasons for drug companies to explore and exploit the potential of this substance that no company could claim as its own. They could make more money promoting proprietary medicines. And doctors could *lose* income by using the nonprescription item which the patient could obtain for self-treatment. Besides, it hadn't been proven up by scientific trials. The evidence of its value was mostly anecdotal (nonscientific). Because of the legal aspects most doctors were content to avoid the use of medicines that lacked scientific backing.

It worked out to be a major serendipity from the establishment's point of view. There couldn't have been a better way to block a cheap substance from replacing expensive proprietaries. Thus it languished in medical limbo yet no one could be blamed for neglecting it. Then Linus Pauling invaded the establishment's turf in 1970 with his book *Vitamin C and the Common Cold* (W.H. Freeman, San Francisco). Whether anyone can be blamed for the interesting exercise in the art of the put-down that followed is left for the reader to ponder.

Pauling declared that 4 to 10 grams of vitamin C,

taken on the first day of a cold and continued the next day if necessary, would offer almost complete protection from the virus. He also allowed that 1 or 2 grams daily might be enough for some individuals while others might need 10 or 15 grams.

The stature of the scientist demanded that the claims be subjected to rigorous investigation and either confirmed or refuted. In the decade that followed, more than 20 scientific trials were conducted which tested various doses of C against a placebo. Most were double-blind—neither the person who conducted the trial nor the one who took the "medicine" knew whether it was C or the placebo until the trial ended.

A few colds may have been prevented by C during the trials but how to know is the problem. What *can* be known is the number of sick days experienced by the C and placebo groups. These indicate that benefits from C ranged from around 20 to 49 percent— which may have included several preventions. But as the results of each trial appeared in medical journals the news media reported only the summaries or the statements of authorities, which did not hype the benefits. And so the public was informed that vitamin C had not been shown scientifically to be of much value in the prevention or cure of the common cold. The negative pronouncements came on almost with the regularity of a commercial, which in effect they were—trashing C.

We have read or heard this verdict ever since— from medical textbooks, FDA publications, health letters, consumer magazines, journal editorialists and various other columnists or commentators. The judgment implies that Pauling and the two physicians, Markwell and Regnier, were wrong. It implies that definitive trials settled the matter.

The fact is that no definitive trial was ever conducted. A proper scientific test of a substance would use the dose regimens which had been reported to be effective. Both Markwell and Regnier had reported such regimens. And Pauling's basic dose of 4 to 10 grams, something of a composite of the other two, offered a third regimen which one would expect to be tested—particularly so, because his claim had initiated the establishment's response.

None of the scientific trials uses those doses. *Not one.*

But what about the Cowan trial in which the dose could have been 4 grams daily, Pauling's basic minimum? Yes, what about it? Why was there no benefit at all? Cowan's first trial showed a benefit from only a half gram daily. All the major trials showed *some* benefit at the 3-gram level. And why were the reactions from C so similar to the reactions of the placebo group? Why was there not one complaint of bowel looseness from anyone supposedly taking that much C? Should we wonder if an error excluded C from the trial altogether? It does seem so. Not only to me. Dykes and Meier in a 1975 review of major cold trials devoted 70 lines to Cowan's low-dose trial. Two of Anderson's trials rated 63 lines. But Cowan's high-dose trial was merely mentioned with 4 lines under the heading of additional studies. Had they too suspected an error?

The daily dose of C used in most of the trials to-taled 3 grams or less. The T.W. Anderson trial reported in 1974 is typical. Of the regimens tried, 3 came close to Pauling's basic 4- to 10-gram schedule but never matched it. They only nibbled at the edges. One regimen started at a gram a day as a continuous dose, taken even before a cold started. This has been termed a *prophylactic* dose. At the start of a cold, 3 more grams were added so that 4 grams were taken for 3 days.

But this method merely confirmed earlier reports that a continuous dose is almost worthless as an additive to a treatment dose. In 1973 Schwartz reported that a group taking 3 grams of C daily for 2 weeks before being inoculated with a cold virus received no more protection than a group taking a placebo. And in 1974 Briggs reported a double-blind study which found that a continuous 1-gram daily intake had no more effect against a starting cold than a 50-milligram daily intake. Drug tolerance appears to develop.

The *rise* in daily dose at the start of a cold is the important factor. Pauling's basic minimum would have been matched only if *all* of the 4 grams had been taken at the start of a cold and continued the following day if necessary. Anderson did use this amount— also an 8-gram dose—but for one day only. The larger dose was seen to be more beneficial but a follow-up trial did not pursue this lead. Lower doses were used instead—even though the results mentioned below had been published in time to allow the abandonment of the low-dose approach.

In 1973 Hume and Weyers reported that a disruptive shift in the white cells of the blood occurs during the first day of a cold. The C content of this component drops sharply, sometimes to the levels seen in scurvy. As mentioned earlier, this drop, and the cold, can be prevented—but a 5-gram *rise* in dose is necessary. Furthermore, the high intake must be maintained for at least 3 days. This agrees with Regnier's recommended 5-gram minimum. The Hume and Weyers subjects actually took 6 grams of C daily but 1 gram was a continuous dose, indicating again that such doses are of little value in treating colds. This holds true even at higher levels. Pauling adds to his 18-gram daily C intake when he feels threatened by a cold virus.

Following the Hume and Weyers paper the Karlowski group "rushed into operation" (their words) a trial which used 6 grams daily—but in a manner that would assure failure (1975). Half of the dose, 3 grams daily, was started in late summer, long before the cold season, allowing ample time for drug tolerance to reduce its effectiveness to near zero, as the earlier reports had already proved. So the *rise* in dose was only 3 grams. Clearly not enough. And it was not taken at the first sign of a cold. It was delayed up to 24 hours, in disregard of all the warnings against delay.

Commentators not familiar with the total picture or not caring to mention that a continuous dose is of no benefit as a cold remedy could then point to a 6-gram regimen as proof that higher doses are no more effective than low doses. No trial afterward corrected the flaw. Since Pauling's book, no 5-gram or even a 4-gram *rise* in dose was ever given at the start of a cold and continued for 3 days in any scientific trial reported. Researchers continued to keep the doses low, perhaps because the road to publication was wide and smooth.

Could it be said that proper dosage had been carefully avoided in all the scientific trials? The arch of an eyebrow needn't subside as we ponder the only other possibility—that the researchers hadn't read the medical literature and didn't know what they were doing. This would label them incompetent, an unlikely tag. It appears that they had studied the literature well and knew exactly what they were doing.

So we see the establishment as having betrayed a trust to look after our stake in the matter. It allowed a full house of anecdotal evidence to be beaten by jokers from a different deck. All in the name of science. This is not to contend that an orchestrated fix occurred. Nothing of the sort was necessary. anyone with good sense knew the odds against publication of a paper highly favorable to C.

And anyone familiar with the extensive medical literature on vitamin C needs no great gift of wisdom to grasp the line of thought behind this monumental snow job. The substance is a major threat to revenue in too many areas of the healthcare system to be allowed scientific recognition as a therapeutic drug for even one condition other than scurvy.

Vitamin C if taken properly would ruin the market for cold and flu remedies and most antiviral drugs as well. Then folks might learn of the many other benefits of high-dose C. The establishment simply cannot afford to let that happen. The snow job fashioned by the cold trials collectively was just one method employed to discredit the effectiveness of C and its advocates.

The facts of life: Many medical journals are owned by publishing companies. The journals would not survive if drug companies refused to support them with ad revenue. Many other journals are published by state, regional and national organizations. They exist to serve their members. Their editors see no benefit to the members in any article that could greatly diminish the need for member services or the profit of their advertisers.

Some journals that carry very little advertising are sponsored by large corporations, including pharmaceutical companies. The arrangement doesn't inhibit publication of favorable studies or anecdotal evidence about the benefits of extra intake of C. But one wonders if large-scale scientific trials which provided conclusive proof of benefit plus legal support when used in therapy would be accepted for publication. Most of the recent articles that supply details of therapy with vitamin C are published in journals which carry no advertising. These are not widely read because their circulation depends on the few subscribers who recognize the problems of advertiser control.

I submitted an article dealing with the antiviral and other properties of vitamin C to two national dental journals. The editors, nondentists, returned it without a dentist ever having read it to judge whether it would be of interest to the profession. A full-page color ad for a proprietary antiviral drug was appearing in each issue of the journals at the time. Plainly, it was not in the magazines' best interest to publish the article. The editors were well indoctrinated in the economic principles of the situation. In other words, ad revenue can be used as a bribe to prevent publication of material which could reduce demand for a product.

Nor is the popular press inclined to allow a questioning of the C-versus-colds verdict. My letters or articles sent to consumer, elderly, health and news-magazines have never been allowed to convey my findings to the readers. Most of the publications of course seek cold-remedy ads. But one wonders whose interest a no-ad consumers publication serves by continuing to denigrate C as a therapeutic substance without at least exploring the issue.

The reluctance of the other editors to set the record straight is more understandable. A long chore of reading in a medical library would be necessary in order to confirm my allegations. Editors wouldn't want to assign a high-priced researcher to the job just because a letter or article, which could have zinged in from a crackpot, claimed that all those scientific tests had failed to use a proper dose regimen. They would simply rely on the advice of their doctors, who would of course stick by the establishment's line rather than strive to contradict it. The doctors would counsel against getting worked up over a few sniffles, particularly when the word is out that high doses of C might be bad for us. Yet the side effects of aspirin are constantly in the news even as articles keep advising it for one ailment or another.

In an attempt to overcome this editorial inertia I offered a bet—a new Cadillac to the first one on the staff of a newsmagazine who could prove me wrong. There were no takers.

Perhaps they wanted a Mercedes. Or perhaps the trots, a common side effect of C when it is taken improperly, had afflicted the editors during personal trials of the vitamin. Probably nothing would have altered their mindset against the "stuff" after such an experience. If that is the sole reason for their bias we are tempted to hope that the stuff had been taken very, very improperly.

3
On Cancer

"Okay," the guy said, "so maybe they threw us a curve when they tested vitamin C against colds. But they did prove it wasn't any good against cancer, didn't they? A couple of times, I heard."

The couple of times the guy referred to are the Mayo-group trials, perhaps. Both received substantial media coverage, probably because Pauling was involved again. Seems like we have a carryover of a fantasy from the Wild West operating here: shoot down a top gun while the crowd stands watching.

Was it a fair fight? You be the Special Investigator. Examine the evidence. Put your finger on the reason why Pauling's study found vitamin C to be of considerable value while two others determined that it was of no benefit. Clues will turn up as we move along.

The mystery begins around 1970 when Cameron, a Scottish surgeon with more than 20 years experience in cancer therapy at the time, decided to give 10 grams (usually) of vitamin C daily to patients having advanced cancer. They had reached the point where they were considered untreatable by any known therapy. This is called terminal cancer.

Cameron admits to being skeptical of the idea at first. But there was a bit of logic behind it so he gave it a try, not expecting much but keeping an open mind. He noticed that after about a week on the dose most of his patients perked up, needed less pain medication and ate better.

Still, most of the patients continued to die. After all, they had untreatable cancer. Usually they felt better on high C for a time then rapidly declined. Cameron noticed that some of them entered this phase when "for one reason or another" the high dose of C was discontinued. He also noticed that the decline could be delayed by increasing the dose. A patient with kidney cancer improved and lived 8 months longer when his intake of C was doubled to 20 grams a day.

Favorable responses of that sort convinced Cameron that high-dose C was indeed beneficial to some cancer patients. The case that provided the best evidence that C is of value involved a man who had a type of lymphatic cancer that is treatable by radiation and chemotherapy. The man had been transferred to the hospital for this regimen but a backlog of work in the radiology department caused a delay. He was started on 10 grams of C daily by the intravenous route as a palliative measure.

Two weeks later when his turn came up for radiation he did not need it. The intravenous C regimen had erased all clinical signs of the disease. Pathologic evidence seen on earlier x-rays had vanished. He was put on a 10-gram oral dose of C and discharged. About 3 months later the dose was tapered off at the rate of 2½ grams per month, reaching zero at the start of the fourth month.

By the end of the fourth month, symptoms of the cancer had returned. The 10-gram oral dose was resumed but failed to do any good. The man was then given 20 grams of C a day intravenously. This regimen again routed the signs and symptoms of the disease in two weeks. The man was put on 12½ grams a day and discharged. Five years later the man was alive and well, working regularly and still taking the daily dose of C. No sign or symptom of the disease was evident.

Over the years Cameron accumulated enough medical records of patients whom he had started on C at the untreatable stage to compare them with the records of other physicians' patients in the same hospital who had not been given extra C. Each of his patients was matched with 10 similar individuals having the same cancer and at the same stage of the disease—untreatable, as noted in the records. In all, 100 C-treated patients were compared with 1000 patients who had received no C other than that supplied by the diet. An evaluation of the data was published in 1976 by Cameron and Pauling. They published a refined version in 1978.

Excluding those who lived beyond the study period, Cameron's patients were seen to survive, on average, 251 days longer than those not on the high-C regimen. Twenty two of them (22 percent) lived beyond a year, averaging almost 2½ years total survival time. Of those 22, 8 were still alive at the end of the study period, 3½ years after being considered untreatable. None of the 1000 non-C patients lived that long. Only 4 of them survived even a year after being judged untreatable.

But remember that this is a retrospective study—a look back at patient records. This type of study is considered vulnerable to bias, no matter how neutral the investigator might strive to be. For example, Cameron could have judged his patients to be untreatable much sooner than other physicians in the same hospital judged theirs to be. Therefore his patients would have been seen to live longer even if they hadn't taken extra C.

An indicator less subject to one doctor's judgment would be the patients' own response to the disease. They all realized they were in trouble on the day they first sought treatment. This first-visit date is not subject to control by a doctor. Cameron and Pauling realized this and compared these dates with patient survival time. They found it made very little difference in the outcome, so there appears to be no distortion of data in that area.

Another area where bias could be a factor is in the selection and matching of C and non-C cases. This was done by employees in the records department who presumably were neutral. Their work was checked by Cameron, however.

Getting suspicious? ... Well, let's kick this thought around: Suppose Cameron, instead of wanting to arrange an unbiased study, decided to make it appear that the vitamin-C treatment was useless. In other words, suppose he decided to equalize the results so that the 1000 non-C patients would show survival times that compared equally with his 100 cases. Since 22 of his cases survived beyond a year he would have had to locate 216 more non-C patients who had lived that long and add them to the 4 who did. And, to compare with his 8 longer-term survivors, 80 of those 220 would need to be living beyond the end of the study period.

Could he have done so? For an answer, one would need to examine the records of the non-C patients who were *not* selected for the study in order to see if that many patients in the files met the requirements. We cannot do so. Therefore, as in many a mystery plot, the matter will be left dangling while we move on—or rather while we digress a moment. Or are we planting a clue?

In 1979 the scientific journal *Cancer Research* published a Cameron-Pauling paper which detailed the reasons for their belief that high-dose C is useful in the treatment of cancer and that moderate doses may be preventive for some types. They mentioned again an observation that they and others had discussed earlier—that abruptly discontinuing a high-C regimen can further weaken a sick patient. It is a jerk-the-rug-out-from-under surprise to the body that can be likened to a drug-withdrawal reaction, only worse.

The reaction has been termed *rebound scurvy*. This describes the C-starved state of the body that had been accustomed to a regular routine of processing large amounts of C. It does not occur when high C is stopped after only a few days on the regimen, however. Healthy individuals may even stop a 2-week high-dose regimen without noticing anything. Schrauzer reported the possibility of a delayed effect, however (1973). As a personal experiment he took 10 to 15 grams of C daily for 2 weeks then stopped abruptly. Some of the signs and symptoms of scurvy appeared 4 weeks later—loose teeth, bleeding gums, muscle aches and rough skin.

The elderly and the sick should be warned against stopping high-C intake so abruptly. In a couple of days they may feel like the fatigue of scurvy will do them in. This reaction hasn't been proved but oldsters needn't wait 100 years for a scientific confirmation. They can experiment personally as my brother and I, both oldsters, have done. Tapering by ½ gram a week is less traumatic.

Back to the case at hand. To test whether cancer patients on extra C live longer, a group at the Mayo Clinic set up a randomized placebo-controlled double-blind trial on such patients. That's about as scientific as you can get with humans—unless they're identical twins. As in Cameron's cases, patients took 10 grams of C a day by mouth until death or until they could no longer take oral medication. Also as in Cameron's cases, several types of cancer were involved. But none of Cameron's patients had had radiation and only 4 had had chemotherapy. All but 5 of the 60 Mayo patients on C had been given radiation or chemo or both. The placebo group was similar.

The results, published in 1979 (Creagan), showed

no significant difference in longevity between the groups. Actually, at any given time more C patients were living than those on placebo except on about 4 dates. In short, the C group outlived the placebo group, even though there were 5 percent more patients on placebo. Not mentioned in the abstract (the summary, the only part which is read by many professionals) is that the C group had better appetite by 13 percent, less pain by 60 percent and twice as many had more strength.

The trial was criticized as not being comparable to Cameron's study because so many patients had been given chemotherapy. This damages the immune system which is considered an aid to high C in cancer therapy. A second trial was then set up, using terminal cancer patients who had not had chemotherapy. Only patients with cancers that had originated in the colon or rectum were chosen because no therapy was deemed to be effective against those cancers at the time. Therefore the patients were not being denied treatment, which would be worthless anyway, just to supply cases for a trial. (So why were more than half the patients who stopped participating in the trial given chemotherapy later? Who paid? Readers may wonder if predation on cancer patients is limited only to quacks.) During the trial they were given 10 grams of C or a placebo daily until they could no longer take oral doses or until they had a 10-percent weight loss or until the disease began to progress markedly.

The results: difference in survival time between the two groups was again insignificant, as in the first trial. But the percent of C patients living at any given time as compared to the placebo group was just opposite to that seen in the first trial. At no time were there more survivors taking C than those taking placebo. In short, the placebo group outlived the C group.

The authors felt that the only difference between their trial and the Cameron-Pauling study seemed to be that looking at medical records to judge high-C therapy introduced a bias which did not occur in their scientifically-conducted trial (Moertel, 1985).

Once more, as after the cold trials, the word went out that Pauling had been wrong. The top gun had been shot down again.

Okay, Special Investigators, start deducing. Why did the results turn out so differently from the Cameron-Pauling study? Ponder a moment. Consider the clues ... Ah-yes, more likely the flaw is in the Mayo-group trial. But not in the type of cancer involved. Cameron's colorectal cancer patients on C fared rather well. One of the 8 who lived beyond the study period had colon cancer.

We must look elsewhere. Notice that in the first Mayo-group trial the C and placebo doses were taken until death or until the patient could no longer take oral medication. This matched the method of Cameron. But notice that in the second trial the doses were discontinued early. Not only were they stopped when patients couldn't take C orally but also when a 10-percent weight loss occurred or marked progress of the disease was evident.

By definition terminal cancer progresses. Supposedly, the trial had been designed to see if high-C therapy would slow this progress. By stopping it early the trial was stripped of its purpose before any effect could become apparent. The trial was useless. Yet the results were accepted for publication in a widely-read medical journal, fed to the media and accompanied by an editorial from an authority in the National Cancer Institute who stated that it is difficult to find fault with the design or execution of the study. Could he not see that jokers from different decks had been dealt in?

Now recall what happens when a high-C regimen is stopped abruptly. The body is distressed, as in scurvy. Anyone at the time who read the medical literature was aware of the reaction. Rhead and Schrauzer discussed it in 1971 and, as mentioned, Cameron saw a rapid decline in health after stoppage of C. Take two moribund patients, equally sick. Start one on a high-C regimen and the other on a placebo. Weeks later, stop the doses on both, abruptly. The one on placebo notices nothing and is no better or worse. But the one on high C suffers from deprival and may die within days.

The effect is made plain by the chart accompanying the results. Two lines, one solid, one dashed, start at the upper left (all living) and drop toward the lower right, showing percent of living in each group at any given time. The C line is the earlier death line all the way, considerably so after the first year.

One can look at the chart of the second trial and conclude that giving the patients high C killed them all earlier. Or a different conclusion might come to mind: that denying them C after they had taken it for weeks killed them all earlier. Take your choice.

Busy professionals who read only abstracts of published papers would never know that those patients had been deprived of high C abruptly when decline was evident. This is not mentioned in the abstract. A number of professionals do read entire articles, however, and some certainly must have realized how the trial had been stripped of its purpose. Why was there no deluge of criticism? Try not to think of the financial aspects of cancer chemotherapy. Or that researchers pursuing other leads wouldn't care to be upstaged by the success of high C. (Later two of the group's authors announced an advance in colorectal cancer therapy similar to what C was tried for.)

But you may want to speculate on how many letters that pointed out the flaw ended up in the journal editor's wastebasket. And speculate on which is more important to the journal's survival, the 56 pages of medical writings or the 97 pages of advertising. Beautiful full-page color ads by pharmaceutical companies mean money. Even someone who has not yet graduated from economic kindergarten can wonder if they mean anything else.

Speculate also on why the results of a Japanese trial with terminal cancer patients were not mentioned in medical journals here or widely publicized in the popular press. Murata and Morishigi compared low doses of vitamin C (4 grams daily) with high doses averaging 25 grams daily. The results were published in 1982, an update of a 1979 paper. Like that of Cameron and Pauling, this was a retrospective study.

The high-dose group experienced a better quality of life and lived an average of 246 days after being judged terminal. The low-dose group's survival time averaged only 43 days. None of the low-dose patients lived beyond 174 days but a third, 18 of 55, on high doses did, averaging 620 days. Three of the 18 were still living at the time the study ended, averaging 1550 days. The cancers (of thymus, breast and uterus) were still there but not progressing. An interesting observation is that some patients took as much as 60 grams of C daily. But as a group, those taking extra-large amounts—above 30 grams daily—did not live as long as those taking 10 to 30 grams daily. We should not conclude that too much C was the harmful factor, however. The aggressiveness of the cancers involved should be considered.

Now speculate on why cancer specialists everywhere don't provide the benefits of high-dose C to their patients. Certainly most of them are aware of at least some of the favorable reports and the logic behind using the substance. Is it because they may feel that patients would start treating themselves if word got out that the doctor was using only a vitamin? And what would concern the doctor more— loss of revenue or that some patients who can't be helped much by C would lose out on better treatment by other means? The latter would certainly happen. To what extent is the big unknown. But ignoring the benefits of C won't provide the answer.

Or is the doctor afraid of litigation if treatment with C should fail to help? It is not an approved drug for cancer therapy. But no approval is needed for treating with large amounts in order to maintain maximum body levels of it. This is not even done. Hospitals rarely determine the C status of the body. Yet every trauma, physical or mental, draws down body stores of C. Cancer patients who have been traumatized by surgery, radiation and chemotherapy have very little body stores left, Cameron reports. So the patients linger on the brink of scurvy, out of C, out of pep and out of luck.

One of these days the litigation may strike from the opposite direction.

If there is still doubt about C being a potent factor in the killing of some cancer cells, a look at two of Cameron's unusual cases should dispel it. A man with numerous metastases of testicular cancer was given 8 grams of C per day intravenously—but only for a day and a half. By that time a metastatic lump in his mouth had disintegrated and was bleeding profusely. He became comatose and died. At autopsy it was seen that the many secondary cancers all over the body were also dead. The body couldn't handle such an abundance of dead tissue hemorrhaging in so many places, particularly in the brain.

In the second case, a man with widely metastatic kidney cancer started a 10-gram oral dose—and again problems occurred within 36 hours. Death 3 days afterward was attributed to a stroke due to sudden disintegration of the cancer metastasis in the brain.

From those experiences Cameron learned to start dosing with only a gram of C, increasing by a gram each day until settling on a steady dose between 10 and 20 grams. This method avoided a recurrence of the above problems.

High-dose C does not retard the advance of every cancer, he emphasized. About one in five continues unchecked. But about half of the patients benefit significantly and a few of those can live on for years. Cameron recognizes the value of all other forms of cancer therapy. The problem is that most proponents of other therapies do not recognize the value of C.

About the logic of using C in the prevention and treatment of cancer: Consider prevention. High intake raises the body stores of C to the optimal level. And higher tissue levels appear to protect against the start of some cancers. As far back as 1948 Goth and Littman found that cancer usually originates in organs that are low in C. The amount of the vitamin in the white blood cells and platelet component of centrifuged blood is considered a good indicator of the body stores of the vitamin, you'll recall. It's termed the leukocyte ascorbic acid content. Krasner and Dymock reported in 1974 that leukocyte C levels were less than the lower limit of normal in 90 percent of cancer patients examined—and very low in 60 percent.

Examples of papers that are usually cited when discussing the role of C in prevention: Schlegel's 1969 report that the formation of chemicals associated with urinary bladder tumors can be prevented by taking a half gram of C 3 times daily; the 1975 report by DeCosse that 3 grams of C daily caused rectal polyps to shrink or disappear in some individuals (polyps can be precursors of cancer); and Romney's 1985 report that women with uterine tissue changes that precede cancer had only half the blood plasma levels of C that were seen in women not having the condition.

Now the rationale for using high-dose C after cancer has started: 1) Again, high intake lifts the patient out of the weary doldrums characteristic of borderline scurvy, prompting all body systems to function better. 2) As an antiviral substance, high-dose C attacks any viral component that might possibly play a role in cancer growth. 3) Cancers make substances that break down body tissues to allow for easy expansion. High-dose C inhibits the production of these substances and also promotes the formation of a dense fibrous barrier to retard the expansion. Cancer cells can't divide and spread if they have no room. 4) The immune system is bolstered by a copious supply of C. Clean-up cells are stimulated to counter any deviation from normal that cancers tend to encourage. 5) The two major hormone factories in the body are the adrenal and pituitary glands. These normally have the highest concentration of C found in the body. High C keeps them on track.

As can be seen by the Japanese study mentioned, Cameron is not the only authority who has reported success with C in cancer treatment. He and Pauling describe more than two dozen examples from other sources. A remarkable case involved a one-inch diameter tumor in the brain of a physician's wife. Two neurosurgeons as well as her husband urgently advised surgery but the prospect of paralysis of the affected arm and leg terrified her. She chose to take 10 grams of C daily instead. About 2 months later she began to improve. About 5 months later a final brain scan showed no evidence of the tumor.

Another case illustrates the value of increasing the dose if all else fails. A man had part of his stomach and the lymph nodes in the area removed because of cancer. His pancreas was left in although the cancer had spread to it. He began taking 12 grams of C daily but 6 months later the lymph nodes in his neck were enlarged and a blood test indicated that the cancer was active. He was hospitalized and began to fail quickly because the daily dose of C was discontinued. His daughter, a nurse, removed him from the hospital, put him on 20 grams of C daily and gradually increased it to 28 grams. The neck nodes and blood test returned to normal. When he had surgery for gall stones 16 months later there was no evidence of the stomach cancer.

In 1982 Hanck reported remarkable results in treating 3 cancers with high C at a unit of the University of Basel in Switzerland. One, a recurrent tumor of the head and neck, regressed after a regimen of 14 grams of C daily. The patient continued to be free of symptoms 2½ years later. Another patient had an inoperable cancer of the bronchus. He was put on 15 grams of C daily, gained back his weight and went back to work. The third patient had a recurrent cancer of the breast, which regressed after a regimen of interferon and high C. None of the patients had radiation or the more toxic drugs used in therapy.

This is not to imply that chemotherapy is of no

value. Dr. Newbold's book *Vitamin C Against Cancer* (1979, Stein & Day, New York) begins with an account of an exhausted lady who dropped out of a chemotherapy and radiation regimen which was countering her aggressive lung cancer. Newbold's high-C therapy brought her back to health, leaving the reader with the good feeling that all would now be right with the world. But page 66 contains a brief mention that the cancer had returned. Perhaps the high C had not treated for cancer as much as it had brought the lady out of the state of near scurvy which the other therapists had let develop.

Most physicians, whether specialists or generalists, seem almost to nurture the blind spot that keeps them from seeing the need to use C even for its basic purpose. And there is not enough public pressure forcing them to change their ways.

But recently there's been an indication that the bureaucracy has pried its eyes open just a little. For the first time ever the National Cancer Institute held a symposium on C and its relation to cancer. For 3 days in September, 1990 experts from the U.S. and Japan presented evidence of the value of C in this area, giving us hope that the establishment can't hold back the dawn much longer.

Preventionwise, North Americans can take hope from a calculation by G.R. Howe (1990) based on the pooled data from a dozen breast-cancer studies. The risk to postmenopausal women would drop by 16 percent if they'd get 380 milligrams of C daily. And by 24 percent if that intake is combined with a drop in saturated fat to less than 10 percent of total calories. The same combination would drop the risk to premenopausal women by 16 percent.

For other interesting cases regarding C and cancer read the book by Cameron and Pauling titled *Cancer and Vitamin C* (1979, Pauling Institute, Palo Alto, CA 94306–2025).

4
History and Hassles

The health history we are taught can cover a subject only briefly—still it is more than we may care to know at the time. It probably sticks in the minds of some of us that an Englishman found a cure for scurvy in limes and from then on the scourge of long sea voyages was banished while British sailors acquired the nickname *limeys.*

Actually, the British naval surgeon James Lind, a Scotsman, used oranges and lemons in his notable experiment in 1747, the results of which he published in 1753. Carpenter states that the terms "lemon juice" and "lime juice" were used almost interchangeably back then, so one can see why limey caught on. Lemony sounds better with detergents and furniture polish.

Lind's experimental proof was not a breakthrough. It had been common knowledge among sailors for generations that citrus could cure scurvy. It seems to be the fate of vitamin C to garner scientific recognition late and to be universally accepted later still. Even after scurvy hit the British navy hard in the 1780s the Admiralty dawdled because of poor advice from some authorities who were not convinced that issuing citrus juice was the best approach to the problem. The Admiralty finally authorized a daily ration of citrus juice in 1795 but the fleet admirals still had to request it.

Carpenter's *The History of Scurvy and Vitamin C* (Cambridge University Press, Cambridge, 1986) cites many examples of the use of citrus prior to Lind's experiment. In 1498 Vasco Da Gama, off the east coast of Africa, sent a boat to bring back oranges for the sick men aboard. A physician writing about scurvy in 1564 advised that it could be cured with oranges and plants such as watercress. In 1593, after a long voyage from England to Brazil, all but 4 of Sir Richard Hawkins' crew were sick on arrival and happy to trade cloth for oranges and lemons. A London ad in 1607 promoted provisioning with the juice of lemons as a remedy for scurvy and by 1661 the Dutch reportedly had 1000 citrus trees at the Cape of Good Hope.

One wonders why Lind had to prove the obvious in the middle of the next century. Then one reads that intellectuals began to ponder the scurvy sickness. They generated so many ideas about causes and cures that they couldn't see the forest for the trees. The babel prompted John Wesley, the preacher and founder of Methodism, to complain in 1747 that men of learning were setting aside experience and forming theories.

This sort of exercise continues today. Although the theoretical approach to selecting therapy is commendable it can lure the unwary onto thin ice when experience is set aside. Some researchers, disregarding voluminous anecdotal and scientific evidence, look upon high C intake as unjustifiable, believing that a gram or less is plenty. Melethil expressed this point of view (1987). He compared the plasma C level measured after a half-gram dose to the levels seen after 1-gram and 2-gram doses and found very little difference. From this data experts fed an equation into a computer and found that taking a 20-gram dose all at once would make very little difference also. This result led him to question the value of high-C therapy.

He didn't take into account the tremendous accumulation of practical experience—or even scientific experience. The scientific report of R. Anderson in 1980, for example, which indicates that normal adults can have a more active immune system when 2 or 3 grams of C are taken daily. This benefit is not seen at lower doses.

By applying data gathered from healthy men to sick individuals, low-C advocates don't take into account the difference in utilization of C by the sick, as reported in a scientific paper by Faulkner and Taylor more than 50 years ago (1937). Although computer searches of the literature don't reach back far enough to point out much of the knowledge gained in prior generations, they do bring up more recent titles which head articles showing that plasma C levels drop in ill health and that high doses can restore the levels.

Also not taken into account is the fact that most

drugs, including high-dose C which acts as a drug, are given in divided doses to maintain high amounts in the bloodstream. One should not make a judgment on the value of C or any other drug with data gathered from a single undivided dose which may leave quickly via the urine. (Some drugs are expelled so quickly that they are given with retardants in order to maintain high blood levels.)

Finally, the study didn't take into account the probability that computer printouts do not necessarily predict with accuracy when living tissue is involved. As the old farmer said of his mules, "You can hit Jack on the butt with a rock and get him to go but try that on Jenny and God knows what'll happen!" So it is with any tissue that is connected to a brain, particularly during sickness. The computer calculated that the gut and kidney interaction would limit the plasma C level to less than 3 milligrams per deciliter, without a "thought" to massive absorption. It saw that a gram or two can provide for the 3-milligram figure, therefore dismissed the value of higher intake. The demands of sickness were completely disregarded by its programmers.

The 3-milligram maximum is off-target also. Some of Cameron's patients were found to have plasma C levels of more than twice that. In 1981 J.D. White reported a fasting level of 17 milligrams per deciliter in a young man who took 15 grams of C daily for 4 months.

According to high-C advocates hereabouts, the only experience some researchers appear to take into account is the better chance of getting published when a negative assessment of C is written.

Long after Lind proved that citrus fruits could prevent and cure scurvy the argument continued over its cause. It was due to copper poisoning, a surgeon suggested, pointing to the use of copper kettles used in preparing food on naval ships. Those sailors were down with scurvy more often than the sailors on merchant ships which used iron kettles. He had a good thought. Copper destroys vitamin C. But of course others could point to the occurrence of scurvy where food did not come in contact with copper.

Mental depression is mentioned often enough in accounts of scurvy that it was thought to be a contributing cause, along with cold, humidity, heat, salt air, ptomaines, etc. A French professor in 1871 pondered what he had seen and decided the only common factor was lack of fresh vegetables in the diet. Another refuted this by noting that Eskimos who subsist mainly on meat are usually free of scurvy—although he admitted that fresh vegetables could cure the disease. But, he argued, quinine cures malaria yet the cause of it is not lack of quinine. He settled on contagion. The germ theory of disease was gaining acceptance and contagious conditions existed during outbreaks of scurvy—people crowded together in armies, navies, prisons and cities besieged.

There were too many reports of scurvy coming on in isolated areas for the contagion theory to gain credence, however. Carpenter recounts the experience of 4 Russian sailors stranded for 6 years on a remote coast of Spitzbergen in the 1740s. They ate raw reindeer meat, a bit of cress called scurvygrass that could be found in small quantities there and 3 of them drank the blood of the killed reindeer. One could not bring himself to do so. He died of scurvy while the rest survived.

The variability of C in concentrated citrus juice fogged the issue also. Much of the C content was lost by boiling the juice to a syrup. Even more was destroyed if copper boilers and piping were used. Further, some expeditions took the weaker lime juice rather than lemon juice which contains 50 percent more C. Limes, being more acidic, were thought to be a better scurvy preventive. Not so. And we now know that some debilitation reported in polar expeditions was due to the lead in soldered cans. Those who assumed that citrus juice was of no value may have confused lead poisoning with scurvy, the mild form. H.N. Holmes in 1939 noted the similarities.

For a century and a half the guessing continued, even after 1900. Carpenter attributes the breakthrough toward learning the cause of the disease to economics, prejudice against the disease-carrying rat and a lucky choice by a Norwegian bacteriologist, Axel Holst. He was trying to solve the problem of beriberi, a disease caused by lack of vitamin B-1. The pigeons used in his experiments weren't satisfactory so he decided to switch to mammals. Dogs were expensive to keep and rats were not the nice mild lab critters we see now. So he chose a common children's pet of the time, the guinea pig—one of the few mammal species which, like humans and other primates, cannot make C internally. But he didn't know that.

He put some guinea pigs on a restricted diet and saw them develop scurvy. He and a pediatrician. Theodor Frolich, who was studying infant scurvy, assured themselves that the affliction was indeed scurvy, in an animal species they considered immune to it, and published their findings in 1907. Interestingly, a group of scientists in the U.S. Department of Agriculture had seen the same degenerative changes in the 1890s but didn't recognize it as scurvy, so missed going down in history as contributors to the solution of the problem.

Carpenter credits the Polish scientist Casimir Funk, doing research in London in 1912, with the idea that rickets, scurvy, pellagra and beriberi could be prevented if four particular substances, one for each disease, were supplied in the diet. Funk suspected that these vital substances were nitrogen compounds called amines—vital amines, shortened to *vitamines*. The terms *nutramines* and *auximones* were also used in reference to these substances for a time.

In the following years other scientists came onstream with papers which detailed their work in the vitamine area. McCollum called his substances *fat-soluble A* and *water-soluble B*—what we now know as vitamins A and B. In 1917 he disagreed with Funk on the scurvy issue. It was not a dietary deficiency that afflicted the guinea pigs, he said, it was merely constipation.

He was wrong, of course, but he was thinking when he proposed the idea. He reasoned that rats didn't develop scurvy on the same restricted diet. And the guinea pig, being more like a rat than a human, would not get scurvy like the human—unless the guinea pig and the human were somehow similar in that respect. He had a 50–50 chance of choosing that alternative but opted for the constipation theory.

Other scientists soon decided that guinea pigs were indeed more like humans in the need for the certain something in the diet that could prevent scurvy. They set about trying to extract it in pure form. But even before that was accomplished they gave it the letter name C. Credit for naming it is given to Drummond but my reading finds that the team of Harden and Zilva first used C in a published paper. The two set up a diet experiment on rats, using the so-called accessory food factors fat-soluble A, water-soluble B and the anti-scurvy factor which they termed, quite logically, the C diet. The year was 1918. In 1919 Drummond, an eminent nutritionist of the time, reinforced this designation by calling the substance *water-soluble C*. In 1920 he proposed that the solubility labels and the last letter of vitamine be eliminated, thus initiating the terminology we now use.

The generic name *ascorbic acid* was arrived at in a more roundabout manner, with humor and hassle attending. The race to isolate the substance in crystalline form was won by a chemist who wasn't even looking for it. Albert Szent Györgyi was studying oxidation-reduction reactions, using the adrenal glands of cattle to supply large amounts of a reactive substance with a powerful reducing capability. He extracted it in crystalline form and found it to be made up of carbon, hydrogen and oxygen in sugar-like proportion. The names of sugar end in *ose*—glucose, sucrose, dextrose, etc. Looking back in 1963 he recalled that he did not know the exact makeup of the molecule. Being ignorant of this, he called it *ignose*. Harden, mentioned above, was then editor of the *Biochemical Journal,* in which the scientific achievement would be announced. He vetoed the flippant idea—and vetoed *Godnose* also. The two scientists then agreed that its name would be *hexuronic acid*.

Szent Györgyi mentioned in the paper, published in 1928, that hexuronic acid could be obtained from oranges also and that it must be an essential part of the "reducing factor" of the juice which had received the attention of students of vitamin C. This is as close as he came to saying it was vitamin C. Later he said he felt it was.

He didn't attempt to try his hunch on guinea pigs but sent a sample to Zilva, who had been working for years to extract the pure crystals. Zilva tested the sample and concluded that it was not C. Other scientists examined the substance. Some suspected that it was indeed the long-sought vitamin and that Zilva had been fooled by the changeable nature of it. That possibility plus a new assistant versed in the ways of the vitamin, Svirbely, rekindled Szent Györgyi's interest in it. Svirbely tested it on guinea pigs and proved it was C. Who did so first became a controversial issue for a time. Two other scientists, King and Waugh, actually beat Svirbely into print by 2 weeks in April, 1932.

In 1933 Szent Györgyi changed the name from hexuronic acid to *ascorbic acid*, thereby involving it in its first sour relationship with the establishment. On reading the medical literature of the middle 1930s one occasionally comes across the term *cevitamic acid* used in reference to vitamin C. The reason can be traced to a report of the Council on Pharmacy and Chemistry of the American Medical Association in the AMA Journal of January 5, 1935.

In the previous year the Council objected to the term "ascorbic" because it was therapeutically suggestive, meaning that it advertised the substance as an antiscurvy medicine. That sort of promotion ran counter to a long-standing official policy which excluded such names from the AMA book *New and Nonofficial Remedies*. Therefore the Council changed the name to cevitamic acid.

Scientists of the world were not impressed by the arbitrary action. The Council members had done no laboratory work to justify the privilege of naming the substance. And because so much of the work was being done outside the U.S. the change was barely recognized. In 1939 the Council faced reality and decided to go with the flow. They entered C in the book as ascorbic acid.

Incidentally, the number of published research papers on C peaked in 1939. The Index Medicus, a listing of papers of interest to healthcare personnel, contains about 750 titles for that year relating to C, about 130 of which were published originally in

English. During World War II the papers dwindled to a trickle. In the last two decades the yearly worldwide count ranges from around 250 to 300. That's more than one every working day to be read if a doctor wishes to keep abreast of all knowledge concerning C alone. To cut the chore down to size, an abridged index is available. Its stated purpose is to provide rapid access to material of immediate interest to the practicing physician.

It is interesting to note that the article which reported the drop in leukocyte C at the start of a cold, and the amount of C needed to prevent it, is not indexed in the abridged volume. Pauling had written an introductory article preceding it. Had this prompted the establishment to omit any reference to the important paper? Or were the antiviral implications reason enough?

After a year of lab work Szent Györgyi had accumulated less than an ounce of crystalline ascorbic acid from cattle adrenal glands, the best source he knew at the time. Harris and Ray reported in 1933 that the adrenal cortex (outer part) has 3 times more C than an equal weight of orange juice. Back in Hungary Szent Györgyi couldn't obtain large quantities of cattle adrenals so had to find another source. He had tested cabbage and other vegetables earlier but not the garden pepper. This he found to be a rich lode. In a few weeks he had pounds of vitamin C. He received the Nobel Prize, in part for the discovery of C, in 1937.

Synthesis of the vitamin was reported in 1933 by the Haworth team in England and the Reichstein group in Switzerland. It was first made from xylose, then more economically from glucose. According to Cathcart the principal source of the glucose today is corn.

5
The Kidney and C

A few individuals should be wary of taking large amounts of vitamin C but the matter needs clarification. When I asked around, the concern most frequently expressed focused on kidney stones. No doubt this is due to warning statements in nearly every medical textbook and popular health publication.

Like all excursions into the realm of the possible each reprinting expands more toward the probable than appears to be warranted. A health magazine in September, 1990 carried an item about researchers who found C to be helpful for lung irritability during colds but they cautioned that taking more than a gram a day may be unsafe for people who develop kidney stones.

Give them credit for directing the caution only to those people who have a tendency to form stones. But dock them several points because, as scientists, they embraced a shred of evidence so tenuous that it is even less than flimsy. A search of the medical literature turns up only a letter to a journal by Briggs in 1973 that a doctor in Africa knew of a man who passed a stone after taking 2 grams of C daily for 2 weeks. And a letter by Roth in 1977 about a man who passed a stone after taking a gram of C a day for "many months."

In a system that functions on scientific evidence the first reaction to such reports is to think coincidence. As Kean reminded readers in a comment on Briggs' letter, only an x-ray showing no stone prior to the start of the C regimen would establish a connection (1974). A more likely probability is that C, being a mild diuretic, caused an increased urinary flow which flushed an existing stone out of the system. As for the second report, Lyndon Smith, a urologist with long experience in treating stone-forming patients, wrote that extra C might possibly be a factor if the intake gets up to 4 grams or more a day.

He cited 5 cases in which that amount just may have tipped the calcium-oxalate balance in stone formers who had been free of stones for a time. Each began taking at least 4 grams of C a day and developed a stone from 1 to 3 years afterward. He stated that stone formation stopped after the high C intake was discontinued (1978).

The account is anecdotal evidence, you know. The type that would be sniffed at as an unsubstantiated claim if an experienced physician reported that high C had stopped a cold in 5 patients. So those who sniff at the anecdotal evidence relating to colds should have difficulty accepting Smith's report, particularly in the cases in which stones did not appear until 3 years after the start of high-C dosing.

A hard-core doubter could argue that those patients would need to be free of stones for 3 years prior to the C regimen in order to compare with the stone-free time while on C. So a patient who was stone-free for a total of 6 years would need to be observed for another 6 years to make sure that a stone wouldn't occur every 6 years anyway. Therefore, 12 years of observation would be necessary in order to establish that the patients would not develop stones every 6 years regardless of the amount of C taken. But high-C dosing was not common before 1970. These cases were reported in 1978. A hard-core doubter would contend that a shortfall existed in observation time.

The reason for thinking that high C might cause calcium oxalate kidney stones arises from the observation that a certain percentage of the C ingested leaves via the urine as calcium oxalate. It was assumed that the more C taken the more oxalate would show up in the urine. But the relationship is not directly proportional. To fuzz up the matter further, some of the tests for oxalate inflate the figures. One testing procedure actually creates oxalate in voided urine (Fituri, 1983). Even delaying the assay of a specimen will raise its oxalate level. Conyers demonstrated this convincingly in 1985. The false high readings led to false assumptions. Newer testing methods have cleared up much of the confusion.

In 1976 Briggs reported finding 3 individuals out of 67 whose urinary oxalate soared after taking 4 grams of C daily for 7 days. No one else has reported such high oxalate figures, raising doubts about the validity of the findings. There was no mention of the testing method used. Usually such reports do so. We can be certain of one thing, however: the 3 individuals reportedly having the very high oxalate levels never had kidney stones. There's no doubt that Briggs would have mentioned it.

In 1980 Butz reported the effect of high oxalate foods as well as high-dose C, up to 6 grams daily, on the blood and urinary oxalate levels in both stone formers and nonstone formers. He used a newer and more accurate testing method for oxalate. His conclusion: although the blood oxalate level rose somewhat in both groups, taking large doses of C would not lead to oxalate stone formation. At a certain level no more oxalate is formed (Hornig, 1981).

A.H. Chalmers came to the opposite conclusion in 1986, expressing the belief that high-dose ascorbate should be avoided by consistent stone formers. So we see that the newer testing methods did not bring everyone into agreement. The interesting observation in the Chalmers report is that stone formers have low plasma C levels. These individuals convert most of the ingested C into oxalate in the gut before absorption occurs. Not enough C is left to keep the blood level at its optimum. When they were given a half gram of C intravenously the stone formers did not pass the expected amount into the urine. The body needed more, so kept more.

It seems that if stone formers shy away from extra C they will find themselves in a peculiar bind—having low plasma levels of it but afraid to take more because some authorities believe that stones may result. They may take comfort in the conclusions of Butz and the observations of Lyndon Smith that up to 4 grams daily appear to be acceptable. More comfort is to be found in the comments of physicians who have treated thousands of patients with high C for many years. Surely they've treated stone formers.

Klenner was a physician with that kind of experience. In 1971 he called the kidney-stone alarm a scare weapon used by critics of high-dose C. He stated that urine flow must be slow and neutral or alkaline before enough oxalate can precipitate out of solution to form stones. And that 10 grams of C daily is both a diuretic which increases urine flow and an acidifier which keeps the urine at about pH 6. Sherry Lewin, who wrote the book *Vitamin C: Its Molecular Biology and Medical Potential* (1976 London, Academic Press), confirms this, stating that oxalate remains in solution at the pH created by ascorbic acid so that less stone formation occurs. (Lyndon Smith stated in 1974 that oxalate can drop out of urine solutions of normal acidity but didn't supply a pH number.)

By keeping the urine acidic, ascorbic acid along with antibiotics and a diuretic actually helps dissolve the struvite type of kidney stone. Gaker and Butcher reported such a case, supported by x-ray evidence in 1986.

Poser in 1972 reported seeing no stone problems in his years of prescribing high-dose C. Cathcart, probably the physician presently having the most clinical experience with megadose C therapy (over 12,000 patients in 15 years by 1986), stated that stones do not occur. They do not even recur in patients who'd had them prior to taking large amounts of C. He believes that high doses help prevent stones by eliminating many infections which can lead to stone formation

Abram Hoffer, another physician who had years of high-dose C experience, put it this way in 1985: "By constant repetition this (stone) idea, based entirely on conjecture has become enshrined as a fact." Later in the year after labeling the stone idea a myth, he wrote: "Soon we will have a massive bibliography of references to authors referring to one another about a theory unsupported by experimental evidence."

Those comments are reassuring, as are the findings of K.H. Schmidt (1981), Fituri (1983), Tsao (1984) and others that the vast majority of people—those with normal kidney function who handle oxalate normally—need not be concerned that high C alone is a factor in stone formation.

At a conference on vitamin C which was held in 1986 (published in 1987) Rivers addressed the stone issue along with other concerns about side effects. A review of the literature led him to conclude that taking large amounts of C, "in the range of 5 grams and greater," will not cause calcium oxalate stones or other problems such as iron overload, higher uric acid excretion or depletion of vitamin B-12 in healthy individuals.

Stone formers may be a mite less than healthy but it appears that extra C is not the hazard it has been made out to be. Stones have been bothering us long before extra C came on the scene. A personal note: I developed a stone before starting a high C regimen but have had none in the 5 years since. Mine can be blamed on water restriction, the typical response to prostate enlargement.

Magnesium and pyridoxine also play a role. Prien and Gershoff in 1974 reported a trial in which oxalate stone formers took 100 milligrams of magnesium oxide (*not* milk of magnesia) 3 times daily plus 10 milligrams of pyridoxine once daily. The 149 patients had 871 stones during the 4½ years prior to the trial. In the 4½ years during the trial they had only 71 stones, better than a 12-fold reduction even though the treatment didn't help some of them. Perhaps the more absorbable magnesium citrate would.

Pyridoxine is vitamin B-6. The amount taken does not exceed that found in many fortified multivitamin pills. Authorities have warned that nerve damage can occur in some individuals if these reasonable amounts are exceeded. The amount of magnesium oxide, 300 milligrams daily, is not excessive. In fact it equals the recommended daily intake for women and is 50 milligrams less than the quota for adult males.

So far, except for stone formation, we've explored the effect of extra C on individuals with normal kidney function. Pru stated in 1985 that the normal kidney can easily handle the excretion of excess C. The weak kidney is another matter. It may have difficulty passing the extra oxalate that extra C leaves in the bloodstream. The problem is exacerbated when C is given intravenously to these individuals. This delivers more of it to the bloodstream than is absorbed by the gut. The oxalate can precipitate out as tiny crystals and, if flow is sluggish, a blockage may occur.

McAllister in 1984 reported that a 70-year-old man with poor kidney function went to a chelation therapy clinic where he was given 2.5 grams of C intravenously during a 5-hour infusion. He developed the typical severe flank pain associated with kidney clog 12 hours later and passed a small amount of blood before the flow stopped completely. A biopsy of the kidney revealed tubule blockage by calcium oxalate crystals.

Also in 1984 R.D. Swartz reported that giving C intravenously may have contributed to oxalate crystals and reduced kidney function in a particular case where a diseased small intestine had been removed. Only a few inches of it remained. The patient was getting all nourishment intravenously, including 1.5 grams of C a day. Kidney function improved when the dose was reduced to 100 milligrams daily. Urinary oxalate is said to rise in proportion to the length of diseased gut. Apparently this is not seen in all such cases, however (J.Q. Stauffer, 1972 and Lynwood Smith's reply). In this case the extra C may have added just enough oxalate to cause a problem.

A single dose of 45 grams of C given intravenously clogged the kidneys of a very sick woman but the manner in which the C was handled may have been at fault. Lawton (1985) commented that the solution of ascorbate may have partially converted to oxalate before it was given. The account raises the question of whether conversion to oxalate occurred prior to giving C intravenously in the other cases reported.

Fortunately, most people take extra C orally rather than by vein. They wouldn't be so apt to have the problems mentioned. But if their kidneys are on the brink of failure or if they are on hemodialysis they should take no more C than the physician advises. Several papers in the literature indicate that the dose of C needs to be adjusted to the amount that such patients can handle.

Some individuals who have had elevated oxalate levels for years may eventually experience bone discomfort due to oxalate deposits. Ott reported a case in 1986 in which a long-term hemodialysis patient—23 years—was found to have microscopic crystals of oxalate in certain areas of the bones. The patient had taken 2.6 grams of C daily for 7 years, beginning in 1976. Whether the C extended his time in fair health is an unanswered question.

6
Other Concerns

As the use of large doses of vitamin C accelerated in the 1970s the list of possible side effects expanded in proportion. Some of the entries were legitimate concerns which needed to be investigated, such as the relationship to kidney stones. Others, as Klenner contended, may have been scare weapons brandished by critics of high-dose C or by vested interests in the status quo. Once expressed, an ill-founded warning may reverberate in the literature for years, giving pause to the prudent individual as effectively as black cats deter the superstitious one.

A brief rebuttal that it ain't necessarily so does little to counter a cautionary statement that high-dose C might upset a body balance of some sort. Better to follow selections from the literature through an appraisal of the caveat to a final verdict in order to develop firm insights which are less likely to be jarred loose by the kind of lore that black cats must endure. This chapter treats several expressed concerns in that manner.

It was known in the 1950s that C destroys a percentage of vitamin B-12 but the matter was of little importance until high-C dosing became widespread. Victor Herbert (not the composer) prompted a closer look in 1974 when he reported destruction of up to 95 percent of the B-12 in a "meal" which was kept at stomach temperature for half and hour after a half gram of C was mixed in. The findings from this simulated meal led him to warn that taking a half gram or more of C is unwise.

Six months later, in 1975, Afroz wrote of checking the B-12 levels in 10 spinal-injury patients who had been taking 4 grams of C daily for 11 months or more. All showed blood levels of B-12 which were well above the low normal. Three patients had levels above the high normal, indicating that C was *not* depleting the vitamin. Herbert commented that the test may have been faulty—or that the three high readers had liver disease.

That same year J.D. Hines reported the B-12 levels of 90 patients who were taking a half gram or more of C daily. All but 3 had levels in the normal range. The 3 with lower levels had been taking a gram or more of C with each meal for more than 3 years. In one, the B-12 level rose substantially after the high C dose was discontinued. Hines then suggested that 2 or 3 percent of those who take large daily doses of C may exhibit a lowering of the B-12 level after a period of time.

In 1977 Newmark questioned the original test method. Two other tests were more accurate, he stated, resulting in readings 5 to 9 times higher than Herbert's. Using an altered test method, then, Herbert reported that 4 of 18 patients who were taking 2 grams of C daily had low B-12 levels. He had not determined their B-12 status before the high-C regimen, however, and did not mention discontinuing the C dose in order to check on whether the B-12 level would rise, as Hines had done.

One of the low-level patients had been on extra C for only a month and a half, suggesting that the problem may have existed prior to the start of the C regimen. This could apply to 2 of the others also because they had been on extra C for only 3 and 5 months respectively. Most of the patients had been dosing for around 20 months, as had the fourth patient having a low level. (The body uses so little B-12 that 3 to 5 years may pass before ill effects are seen in normal individuals.)

In 1980 after extensive tests Marcus reported that at body temperature B-12 is "completely unaffected" by C in concentrations as high as 100 milligrams per deciliter of fluid, either in food or blood plasma. Since the normal C content of human plasma is around 1 milligram of C per deciliter the threat of its depleting the body of B-12 appears to be nil. The finding by Hines that the B-12 level of a patient rose after high C was discontinued has not been duplicated. In fact Hines wrote Marcus that he found no more low B-12 levels in a later check of patients who were taking up to 10 grams of C daily.

In 1980 Hogenkamp looked over the literature and concluded that at boiling temperature high C can destroy a percentage of B-12 but not all of it because some forms are resistant. A high-C regimen might possibly be detrimental only to rare individuals with errors in B-12 metabolism. In 1981 Ekvall joined the growing body of scientists exonerating C by reporting that 20 children taking roughly 1.5 grams of C daily for 2 years on average (one more than 8 years) were not significantly different from a control group in B-12 levels. She also was informed by Hines that his later investigations found no evidence of C lowering B-12 levels. Her conclusion: it is highly improbable that megadose C would lower B-12 levels in humans.

W.S. Watson's report in 1982 practically settled the issue. Radiotracer techniques were used to follow ingested B-12 to its destiny in both normal individuals and those subject to pernicious anemia. This disease is treated with B-12 and a necessary absorption substance present in normal gastric juice. Watson found that the B-12 in food binds so quickly and firmly with the gastric-juice substance that C cannot affect it. Nor is high C in the body a problem after B-12 is absorbed.

So we see that a poor test method on a simulated meal which was never in a stomach raised a red flag which continues to wave in many recent medical textbooks. Ah-well . . . Nobody got hurt and everybody learned something and in another decade the nonexistent hazard will be deleted from all medical books.

For trivia lovers, ponder the question of why the body needs to ingest B-12 when bacteria in the human intestine synthesize it? Answer: the bacteria which make the vitamin are too far down the line from the stomach's necessary absorption substance, therefore this "homemade" vitamin cannot be absorbed. Dietary lack of vitamin B-12 is very rare but has been reported in true vegetarians who have eaten no meat, eggs or dairy products for years. (Such diets do not include the root nodules of legumes where bacteria produce it.)

As mentioned, the body uses very little B-12. Tissue stores of it will last 3 to 5 years after the stomach is surgically removed, which of course removes the source of the absorption substance. Some years ago I read that a group of true vegetarians had managed to stay healthy for years without having any visible source of B-12. Investigation revealed that insect and mouse-pellet contamination of their food was supplying all the B-12 they needed. The source of this information is beyond recall.

As advocates of High C might characterize it, another round in the struggle to indict the practice as a hazard, or at least a nuisance, opened when H.B. Stein reported in 1976 that a single 4-gram dose increased the amount of uric acid in the urine. More uric acid stones might develop, it was thought, plus gouty symptoms in those who are predisposed to the disease. Distortion of a test for uric acid added a nuisance effect.

The discomfort of gout is due to urate crystal deposits in joints and elsewhere. It is associated with a high blood level of uric acid. Drugs are given to reduce this level, which of course increases the uric acid content of the urine. When such drugs are first started, gouty symptoms sometimes increase. Stein suggested that high C might precipitate these symptoms also.

After publication of Stein's paper Del Arbol wrote that 13 years before, in 1963, he had given a half gram of C intravenously to 6 individuals and noticed increased uric acid excretion by 5 of them. A more extensive intravenous study was reported by L. Berger in 1977. (Doses in the vein eliminate individual differences in gut absorption so that blood levels of C are more easily controlled.) He found that extra C had a mild tendency to increase uric acid excretion in both gouty and nongouty individuals.

K.H. Schmidt's 1981 paper on oxalate, mentioned in the previous chapter, also reported the effect of C on the excretion of uric acid. When 4 persons took 10 grams of C a day for 5 days he saw no change in the rate of excretion. Mitch reported in the same year that both 4- and 12-gram doses caused no significant change in the blood or urine levels of uric acid in 6 nongouty subjects. He stated that if a test method is used which is not specific for urate the readings will show a false high. Fituri reported that blood and urine urate levels were not changed significantly when 8 nongouty subjects took 8 grams of C daily for 7 days (1983).

Thus the uric-acid alarm failed to make big news and faded rather quickly. No documented case of gout flare-up due to high C turned up. But delving into the matter was not without a reward in the trivia category: Besides humans and their primate cousins, the only other animal known to develop urate stones is the Dalmation dog.

About iron: Animal-tissue iron in food is called *heme* iron. It is readily absorbed by the gut. All other food iron is *nonheme* iron. It is not so readily absorbed, yet it is our major source of iron. The vitamin C present in food (or taken with food) increases the absorption of nonheme iron. The C taken with one meal does not increase absorption from later meals. To aid in iron absorption, C must pass through the gut along with the food.

Would a person taking high C for a long time become overloaded with iron? J.D. Cook stated in 1977 that nonheme iron absorption is directly proportional to the amount of C present "over a range of 25 to 1000 milligrams." But he believed that the normal gut would regulate the amount of iron retained by the body so that it would not be a problem except for those who have errors in iron metabolism.

To find out, he gave 9 healthy adults 2 grams of C daily for 2 years. Discussing the results in 1984 he stated, "The surprising finding in this study is the negligible effect vitamin C had on iron stores . . ." It's good news, then, for anyone with normal iron metabolism.

But even the normal digestive system can be overwhelmed by heavy iron intake over many years. A prime example was seen in the adult Bantu living near Johannesburg who had scurvy due to excess iron in the tissues. Where did they get it? The children did not have either condition. Just the adults, mostly males, the heavy beer drinkers. They were brewing their beer in iron kettles which loaded the beer with iron and in turn loaded the drinkers—up to 100 milligrams of iron a day from that source alone. It's 10 times the recommended amount.

The intestinal regulatory system couldn't cope with so much iron. Over the years the body became overloaded, which led to the destruction of vitamin C, with resultant scurvy. Low plasma levels of C are found in all types of iron overload (Lynch, 1967; Wapnick, 1969).

Patients with the hereditary anemias become overloaded with iron from 2 sources. First, in these anemic states the gut takes up more iron as a compensating reaction. Second, iron enters the system via regular red-cell transfusions (R. Propper in Nienhuis, A.W. 1979). A. Cohen suggested in 1981 that these individuals might be better off with low C levels in order to minimize the reaction between C and the excess iron. The two substances have both a beneficial and a detrimental relationship. C is beneficial in some conditions such as when more iron needs to be absorbed and, oddly enough, when more iron needs to be removed from the body by chelation treatments. But in aiding the iron removal the extra C interacts with it to the detriment of the tissues. Walter Henry, in Nienhuis' 1979 paper, tells of a case: A patient with a hereditary type of anemia (thalassemia) developed progressive heart failure and it was assumed that the course would continue downhill. Surprisingly, the heart improved. A careful review of the records revealed that the patient had been started on a half gram of C daily shortly before the heart trouble began and improvement was seen after C was discontinued.

Nor was this the only case. In 8 of 11 patients getting chelation treatment, heart function deteriorated after a half gram of C was given daily. Function improved in 6 of them after C was discontinued. Perhaps the other 2 improved also. The following report suggests that bouncing back may take more time in some individuals. Rowbotham in 1984 reported a similar case involving iron in heart tissue of a man having a hereditary type of anemia due to red-cell destruction which resulted in excess iron deposits. The man had taken a half gram of C daily for 3 years, then a gram daily for a fourth year. He was diagnosed as having congestive heart failure due to excess iron, which was removed by chelation. The extra C intake was stopped. (In this case, extra C was of no value in the chelation treatments.) Heart function had not improved 9 months later but a follow-up report by J.H.N. Bett in 1985 mentioned considerable improvement at 17 months. Pestell wrote that 4 grams of C daily led to heart trouble after 150 transfusions had caused iron overload in a man with lymphoma (1987).

Apparently not all types of iron overload affect the heart. In the Bantu, certain cells in the liver and spleen gathered most of the iron. Some went to the pancreas but the heart was spared of heavy deposits. People who have the hereditary anemias may be more at risk. The reaction to extra C in individuals with sickle-cell anemia is of a different nature and comes on more quickly. In 1971 M.L. Goldstein reported that a woman with the disease had managed fairly well until she began taking extra C to ward off colds. How much was not stated but each time she took a large amount a typical crisis followed. It's due to copper in the cells (E.J. Calabrese 1982).

So it appears that any individual having one of the hereditary anemias or an iron overload of any sort should learn the nature of the problem and the cautions before considering the start of a high-C regimen. Those having the iron-deficiency type of anemia are not in this category. In these cases C is an aid to absorption.

In 1971 G. Rosenthal reported the case of a 52-year-old nurse who'd had a blood clot in a lung and signs of clots in the veins of the calf. The doctor injected heparin anticoagulant initially and switched to an oral warfarin dose on day 9 while phasing out the heparin. On day 17 she left the hospital, stabilized on a maintenance dose of warfarin. Four weeks later the anticoagulant appeared to be losing its effect. The dose was doubled, then almost tripled.

Had she begun taking other drugs or loaded up on foods high in vitamin K, the doctor asked. She said no. But during further questioning she mentioned that she'd been taking extra C each morning as a cold preventive. She had not considered it to be a drug. The amount was not stated but 2 days after stopping the extra C its effect on the anticoagulant therapy had almost vanished. Animal studies had revealed earlier this tendency of C to block the effect of warfarin. But studies on humans have been contradictory.

In 1972 R. Hume wrote that his group had given a gram of C daily for 2 weeks to 5 patients who were on long-term warfarin therapy. This amount of C did not interfere with the anticoagulant action. In 1975 Feetam reported that C doses up to 10 grams a day for 7 days made no difference in the anticoagulant effect of warfarin on humans.

But in 1972 Edgar C. Smith reported that a 70-year-old woman who had left the hospital 6 weeks earlier on an adequate dose of warfarin was admitted again suffering from clotting problems. The dose of warfarin had to be raised 5-fold in order to do any good. The woman had started taking 16 grams of C daily.

So we have 2 case histories and 2 trial studies from which we can draw opposite conclusions. Perhaps the experimental studies ended too soon. Feetam did report that a 40-percent drop in the plasma level of warfarin occurred during the high-C dosing. In the case histories the problems did not develop until 4 or more weeks had passed.

Any individual taking "blood thinner" who reads about the above reports should make a mental note not to start a high-C regimen without having a physician monitor its effect on the anticoagulant. By itself, C is a moderate anticoagulant but apparently in some individuals it reacts with warfarin to produce just the opposite effect.

Another reaction to high C intake involves destruction of the red cells in individuals who have the G-6PD enzyme deficiency. The condition is found in 11 to 15 percent of U.S. black males and about 1 percent of black females. It is also found in a small percentage of other individuals having genetic roots in the ancient "malaria belts" of Africa, around the Mediterranean Sea and eastward to include southern China where about 6 percent of the males are affected. Those having the deficiency are not as incapacitated by falciparum malaria because at one stage in its life the little parasite needs the enzyme in order to thrive in the red cells. This adaptation which was so beneficial long ago can now be a problem.

There are varying degrees of the deficiency as well as different types of it. One type, more prevalent in the Mediterranean area, is the cause of favism, a reaction precipitated when fava beans are eaten. If the degree of sensitivity is quite high, even inhaling the pollen from the plant causes massive destruction of red blood cells.

Vitamin C is so far down the list of drugs which are apt to cause a crisis in G-6PD deficient individuals that it is seldom mentioned. The antimalarial drugs, sulfas, certain antibiotics, phenacetin and viral attacks are among the common causes. But mild red-cell destruction has occurred after oral C doses as low as a gram and half were taken by volunteers having a severe lack of the enzyme, according to Brewer's 1967 WHO report.

So the threat is hardly worth a headline except that this is an inherited deficiency. And in the game of gene roulette at conception a fetus may end up far more deprived of the enzyme than either parent. This was demonstrated in California where a Chinese baby died of massive red-cell destruction 2 hours after birth. The mother had taken up to 500 milligrams of C daily for 2 weeks before delivery.

But she had eaten a few fava beans also (W.C. Mentzer, 1975). In view of the powerful action of fava beans, the amount of C in a quart of fresh orange juice every day may not have mattered. Nevertheless, this should alert couples who have the at-risk background that the pregnant woman's extra C intake just prior to delivery may create a hazard for the newborn when it is suddenly disconnected from the mother's clearance mechanism. The destruction of red cells creates a jaundiced condition which can lead to complications if severe enough. In 1979 Karayalcin reported on this hyperbilirubinemia in a group of black infants and ruled out all possible causes except G-6PD deficiency in conjunction with high plasma C levels in the babies.

Except for the rare individual having almost a complete lack of this enzyme, taking extra C would cause no problem that could be blamed on the deficiency. But intravenous doses should not be given until a test for G-6PD is done. In 1975 G.D. Campbell reported that a man with a burned hand was given 160 grams of C intravenously in 48 hours. His G-6PD status was not determined prior to this "therapy." He died of massive red-cell destruction.

As mentioned, for the Third Conference on Vitamin C Rivers reviewed the literature to arrive at his conclusions on the safety of high doses taken by healthy individuals. He expressed no concerns, even in the area of *systemic conditioning*. This has been discussed earlier but not by that name. It is the reported adjustment the body makes as it becomes accustomed to handling large amounts of C on a regular basis. Because of this adjustment the body suffers a deprival reaction when the dose is stopped abruptly. Those who take high C don't develop a craving for it, therefore they are not addicted. But they do suffer withdrawal reactions.

Rivers didn't think so. He felt that the conditioning effect had not been proved and is not supported by good evidence in the literature. He did not feel that abruptly stopping a high dose would lead to scurvy. In his conclusion he added the "in healthy individuals" qualification. Since those who take high C are said to be a bit daft by opponents of the practice, a healthy high doser probably doesn't exist. So Rivers is well protected against nitpickers. But is he right?

Others think he is wrong. A number of observations on body reactions to the stoppage of high-dose C have been reported. Enough to support a statement that systemic conditioning does in fact occur. Scientists have difficulty accepting anecdotal reports about conditioning or any other alleged body reaction because they've been led astray too many times by the variables which are not controlled as in scientific studies. Nevertheless they do accept a number of anecdotal observations without question. The evidence pointing to systemic conditioning is strong enough to be accepted also.

An abrupt stoppage of high C needn't cause scurvy to signal that the body is distressed. Other effects of low C kick in before that condition becomes evident. The signs or symptoms of subclinical scurvy are varied and may not be recognizable as being due to low plasma C. In 1971 Rhead and Schrauzer reported some observations gleaned from various sources which suggest that conditioning occurs. For example, when the Germans besieged Leningrad during World War II more scurvy was seen in the Russians who had been taking extra C but couldn't get it when supplies ran out. The conditions imposed by the war came close to those that would be set up for a controlled trial. Then there was the Swede who drank large quantities of juice while working the Florida citrus groves. After he quit and went back to Sweden he developed scurvy.

Schrauzer and Rhead reported a scientific study in 1973 which also supported the conditioning idea. Rivers did not refer to it. Part of it contained subjective evidence which may have been considered unsuitable in a scientific paper. The Tsao and Salimi report of 1984 provides more convincing evidence of conditioning. A woman took 10 grams of C daily for 2 weeks then dropped to 125 milligrams a day. Urinary excretion of C after the drop was used as an indication of body reaction. Excretion of C dropped sharply from the above normal readings seen during the high dosing. It reached normal during the second and third day, stayed in the normal range for 5 days then plummeted to near zero. Excretion was zero on day 10. The readings lingered there for 3 days then slowly climbed, entering the normal range at day 18, having been below that for 10 days.

The measurements suggest that for about 3 days the body was so much in need of C that it held onto

practically all of it. This occurred even as it was being supplied with at least 125 milligrams of C daily
in juices plus whatever else was in the diet. The time
when urinary excretion of C was at zero could appear to be a window of vulnerability to attack by an
infectious agent or an opportunity for the advance-
ment of an ongoing disease.

The study also pointed up the difference in individuals. A second woman took the 10-gram daily
dose for 6 weeks but the C excretion, although dropping to low normal after the high intake was discontinued, did not drop lower. Individual differences
can make some claims seem far-fetched. Perhaps
they are not. In Schrauzer's 1973 report he wrote of
taking 10 to 15 grams of C daily for 2 weeks then
stopping abruptly. Symptoms of scurvy came on 4
weeks later and bothered for 10 days before he raised
his C intake. He described the symptoms as classical:
bleeding gums, loosening of teeth, muscular pain
and roughness of skin.

A quite convincing piece of evidence that systemic
conditioning occurs was noted in the chapter on cancer, in the results of the second Mayo-group trial.
In that trial the patients on high C were deprived of
it abruptly. The chartlines show that at no time did
the percentage of survivors in the C group exceed
the percentage of survivors on placebo. Let the
bookies quote the odds against that happening without an influencing factor. We're interested in the factor itself: systemic conditioning. One should always
consider it when taking high doses of C.

As mentioned, it would be easy for anyone to experience a personal response to an abrupt halt of a long-term high-C dose but it seems unwise. Better to take the advice of physicians who have worked with it for years. They all advise a tapering off from high doses. In research experiments scientists often allow 2 to 4 weeks for bodies to adjust before conducting a trial at a different dose level. This implies a recognition of systemic conditioning. If body adjustment is important in research it should be considered important to maintaining good health.

Raising or dropping the dose abruptly during a viral attack is not the same situation, however. The body is in no need of 100 grams a day when diarrhea occurs. A 20-gram drop might be necessary. But if one has been taking 10 or 15 grams a day for months, tapering by a half gram a week or two is the prudent thing to do.

The reason for this long dwell on the subject of systemic conditioning is that it may set up the greatest hazard of all to anyone taking high doses of C: the abrupt deprivation of it during emergency hospitalization. At a stressful time when it is needed most it may not be given, particularly if the physician is not aware of the high intake and the possible complications that deprivation can cause. Or if the physician holds the opinion that systemic conditioning doesn't exist.

Cathcart in 1981 urged those who take high C to carry wallet cards or wear bracelets informing healthcare personnel of the daily dose. Except for a shield against bias, then, the individual would be prepared for an emergency. Maybe he or she would luck out and be attended by a doctor who would even raise the dose to compensate for the demands of stress.

Those who insist that conditioning doesn't occur should forget about animal studies and low-dose, short-term human trials. Just take 10 grams of C a day for a couple months, fellas, then stop abruptly. Sooner or later you'll think you've been run over by a truck. You may even venture to guess the weight of it. The older you are the heavier it will seem.

By now we realize that at a certain level of higher intake C begins to act like a drug and in this capacity it can cause side effects as do other drugs. Even so its safety record would be difficult to beat. To put the issue in perspective it may help if we compare C with two other frequently used drugs, aspirin and penicillin.

In the Abridged Index Medicus, during the decade of the 1980s, the number of entries in the "adverse effects" section under aspirin total 199. For all the penicillins, which are controlled by prescription and therefore subject to more judicious use, the total for the same period is 88. The C tally for the 10-year period is 14. It is not a precise gauge, not a record of every untoward happening but does make for a rough comparison of relative harmlessness.

Nobody has ever been killed by self-dosing with C as has occurred with aspirin. Patients are still suffering fatal reactions to penicillin in spite of all the precautions taken. According to the 1990 Statistical Abstracts of the United States, accidental deaths involving drugs in medicine for the latest year available, 1986, totaled 4187. If C accounted for any of those the dose would not have been self-administered. For so versatile a substance it is remarkably mild.

But keep in mind that those on anticoagulants; those with poor kidney function or on dialysis; and those who have had many blood transfusions or are otherwise likely to have iron overload should take only the amount of C prescribed by a physician. Individuals who have had part of the upper bowel removed should seek the advice of a physician also. The possibility of G-6PD deficiency should be considered during pregnancy by couples with the genetic background.

The nuisance effects of high C should be mentioned also. An excess amount in the urine can distort certain medical tests if the method used is not specific for the substance being evaluated. Testing methods have been improved recently so that the problem is not the headache it once was. But the person being tested should always tell the doctor and laboratory how much C is being taken

A woman of my acquaintance had been taking several grams of C daily but found it inconvenient while on a trip lasting about a month. Back home again, she began to feel poorly and developed edema in the legs. A treadmill test indicated that she had a slight heart problem, prompting the doctor to prescribe an appropriate drug.

She had resumed the high-C regimen and the edema was slowly vanishing. After hearing about systemic conditioning and seeing photos of leg edema caused by scurvy she began to wonder if the laxity in taking high C had caused all the problems. She gradually reduced the heart drug. When she found it made no difference she told the doctor that she now felt better without it, leaving him somewhat puzzled about the nature of the recovery.

There is no proof that lack of C initiated the chain of events or that resuming the high dose rectified sickness but the evidence is suggestive. It also points up the nuisance value in such dosing. Once it is started on a long-term basis it must be continued daily. Haphazard compliance with a schedule will lead to unsatisfactory results. In short, one becomes a slave to it.

The following chapters should help explain why people are willing to do so.

7
The Forgotten Period

The years from 1930 to 1970 could be called the forgotten period with respect to vitamin C. Those were the years before Pauling sparked a renewed interest in it. So much that was learned then has now been learned again—but the knowledge is still being ignored. We can sharpen our perspective by exploring the medical literature of this time.

The first oral use of pure vitamin C to cure scurvy was reported by Sir Leonard Parsons, a British physician who diagnosed a baby as having the disease. From May 22 to June 5, 1933 Parsons gave the infant a total of 450 milligrams of C, said to be as much as is found in 17.5 ounces of orange juice. Today's nutrition manual indicates that about 30 ounces is the equivalent.

In 1918 Hess and Unger reported that they boiled orange juice, neutralized its acidity and injected it into the vein of a guinea pig to cure it of scurvy. Knowing of it, on May 23, 1933 Paul Schultzer, a Copenhagen physician, dissolved 40 milligrams of pure C in a saline solution and injected it into the vein of a man who was down with scurvy. Thus began therapy with the pure substance.

Soon C was being tried on every disease in the book. Many physicians reported good results. There were astute observers among them. Even then they knew what high-C advocates are trying to make us understand today, that the body needs more of it when sick. J.M. Faulkner in 1935 stated: "The observation that infections predispose to scurvy is well established and has led to the suggestion that under these conditions the metabolic demands for vitamin C may be much increased. Our results suggest that these demands are not met by diets heretofore considered adequate so that in infectious diseases relative vitamin C deficiency develops and may constitute a secondary complication of some importance."

Abbasy reported in 1937 that whenever tuberculosis or rheumatoid arthritis flares up the normal daily urinary excretion of C drops off sharply, indicating that the body is mustering all the vitamin it can get hold of. Extra C should be given to make up for this, he stated. Finkle found that many hospital patients excreted much less C than is normal and when given 100 grams intravenously the body kept nearly all of it (1937).

If some practitioners held the opinion that C was a wonderful new drug others felt that it merely rescued the sick from the brink of scurvy so that the body could cure itself. Long experience with the substance was lacking. Theories were more plentiful and doctors were understandably cautious about giving too much of a substance that was considered a vitamin. As mentioned earlier, they didn't know that their Irish ancestors had been thriving on a gram a day.

In the 1930s, although intravenous doses of a gram of C per day had been given to humans for periods of several months, and 10 grams in single treatments (I.S. Wright, 1938), 100 milligrams was still considered substantial. A physician trying it for skin diseases referred to 200 milligrams as a large amount. Another reported discontinuing an "excessive" dose of 300 milligrams. It appears that most physicians believed that extra C could merely restore the vitamin lost during sickness, not act as a medicine.

But a few thought otherwise. Jungeblut, you'll remember, had reported the effectiveness of C against polio virus in 1935. That same year he and others reported that C inactivates the toxins of diphtheria and tetanus. (Jungeblut noted in 1937 that Inamura had inactivated tetanus toxin in 1929 with ovarian follicular fluid which was later found to be rich in C.) Dainow, also mentioned earlier, reported successful treatment of herpes in 1936. Ormerod, citing success by Otani in treating whooping cough, confirmed this in 1937.

The early researchers also knew that C bolsters the immune system. In 1937 Madison and Manwaring reported that it stimulated antibody production in rabbits. In 1938 Eecker reported a correlation between plasma C and the immune response in guinea pigs. And Chu reported that this applies to humans also.

For every positive report, however, one can find

a negative. This prompted Wright to comment in 1938 that the literature was a "mass of material made up of truths, errors and debatable questions, of which the last mentioned group constitutes the major portion." Reflecting on the manner in which the cold trials were conducted in the 1970s, one might suspect that the same incentive to discredit C existed in the 1930s also. The pharmaceutical-medical complex had become aware of the tremendous potential of prescription antibiotics by then. The first sulfa drug had come on the market—and although it clogged up the kidneys unless plenty of water was taken, it promised great therapeutic and financial benefit.

Another factor which tended to discourage the use of high C is that urinary excretion of it rises considerably when the tissues are said to be saturated—but this begins before the body is "brim full." It led to the assumption that the body couldn't use any more. So the early consensus formed that a daily intake of more than a gram and half simply means the flushing of wasted C down the drain. We still hear that high-C users gain nothing but lose "the most expensive urine in the world." A urologist told me as much 5 years ago. But 2 years later he had changed his mind. He had mentioned to a colleague that this fad of taking too much C was getting ridiculous—then he learned that the other urologist was taking 15 grams a day.

It is all the more amusing in view of the fact that the kidneys also flush away many antibiotics quickly, creating a much more expensive urine. Yet smaller doses are not effective. Retardants are given with some antibiotics in order to slow the elimination process. Kiester noted in the November, 1990 *Smithsonian* that when penicillin first came into use it was quite scarce. And because more than half of it was quickly eliminated unchanged, the best way to conserve it was to collect the patient's urine, remove the drug and reuse it.

Apparently the parallel between C and antibiotics was not recognized, either in dose requirements or rapid clearance from the bloodstream. Many researchers therefore continued to use small amounts, sometimes merely as supplements to the diet. Hare, for example, reported in 1938 that rheumatoid arthritis patients improved when 400 milligrams of C was taken in that manner.

Several studies were done on rheumatoid arthritis in the 1940s, using a gram of C intravenously or intramuscularly along with a cortisone compound. Dramatic improvement was seen in some cases but the benefit usually lasted only a few hours and the side effects led to discouraging reports. The reactions appear to have been due to the cortisone preparation, not C. Massell avoided use of cortisone and in 1950 reported giving oral doses of a gram of C 4 times daily for as long as 26 days to 7 patients ranging in age from 5 to 18. The case histories support his conclusion that 4 grams a day was beneficial to the young patients.

From such reports we can track the progression to the use of larger doses. A few maverick physicians found by experience that such amounts were benefi-

cial and went on to record interesting results. Klenner's papers are a good source of these. He was no
dummy; a Phi Beta Kappa with a masters degree in
biology, he was a teaching fellow in chemistry while
studying for a doctorate in physiology when he
switched to medicine.

In 1948 he reported on 42 cases of viral pneumonia
treated in the previous 5 years. The adult doses were
a gram intravenously or in muscle every 6 to 12
hours. These routes had been shown to more than
double the effectiveness of the same dose taken by
mouth, so the equivalent oral dose would be more
than 4 to 8 grams of C a day.

In 1949 he reported treating 60 polio cases during
an epidemic. Intramuscular doses for children ranged
as high as 1 or 2 grams every 2 to 4 hours around the
clock, fever and age determining the dose. Oral
equivalents in these young patients could be higher
than 48 grams a day. Usually the patients were well
in 3 days but after 3 patients relapsed he continued
treating with a gram or two every 6 hours for the
next 2 days. None of those he treated were crippled
afterward. It is unfortunate that a girl in his neigh-
borhood was cared for by another physician who did
not use C. She ended up in braces. A polio case
Klenner treated more than a year later had been para-
lyzed in both legs for over 4 days. The 5-year-old
girl began to improve after the first shot of C and in
a couple of weeks was back to normal (1951).

The shingles cases responded to high-dose C in
short order also. Pain stopped within 2 hours in 7 of
8 patients who were treated with 2- to 3-gram injec-

tions every 12 hours along with a gram orally every 2 hours. The eighth patient, a diabetic, did not experience complete pain relief and required twice the injections because the healing period was twice as long (1949). Those who are concerned about the safety of high C tend to use too little and discontinue the dosing too soon. A retired physician friend advised his friend who had developed shingles to take 5 grams of C daily by mouth. This helped but the man discontinued the dose too soon and suffered for months from the aftereffects that shingles can inflict.

Another case related by a nurse had a happier ending. The victim of severe shingles learned from physicians at a hospital that he could expect a long painful recovery period. He said he had heard about a doctor in the area who treated with C. The hospital staff scoffed at such therapy but he saw the physician anyway and was cured within a week by intravenous infusion of C.

After so many reports attesting to the value of proper dosing with C one must marvel at the reluctance of healthcare personnel to look into its potential. It is not a newly emergent trait in the professions. In the days when advocates of antiseptic procedures were saving mothers from "childbirth fever" obstinate doctors who scorned the practice watched their patients die by the wagonload.

But there is a modern reason for this obstinance in regard to C: the system can make no money from it. Healthcare is big business with all the incentives and competitiveness of big business. The incentives are good in that they've led to the discovery of wonderful drugs. But when incentive and competition replace morality they become hazardous to our health. We've all seen television segments showing how the pharmaceutical-medical complex pushes certain drugs; about the freebies offered to new doctors; about the continued use of a post-heart-attack drug that is 11 times more expensive than a safer and equally effective drug; about the faking of test results and other frauds committed by drug companies; and about the 4-fold increase in x-rays prescribed when doctors have a financial interest in that department. The sooner we realize that the system is not peopled entirely by innocent lads operating on scout's honor the better off we'll be.

Then there is mindset. Klenner in 1951 wrote: "Many physicians refuse to employ vitamin C in the amounts suggested because it is counter to their fixed ideas on what is reasonable; but it is not against their reason to try some new product being advertised by an alert drug firm." This mindset includes the feeling that to treat with C smacks of quackery. The phony operators on the healthcare fringe have peddled vitamins as the cure-alls for whatever ails us so that legitimate physicians find it difficult to do so even when necessary.

In contrast to the conventional bias, McCormick's paper in 1952 called C a chemotherapeutic agent, indicating how far the reasoning of some authorities had advanced in the 19 years since it was first produced in quantity. He wrote that a single injection of C rapidly overcame the toxic effects of a scorpion sting. Klenner also reported on the value of C for snake or spider bites as well as for anaphylactic reactions. A little girl in a coma from a black-widow spider bite was started on 4 grams of C intravenously along with some calcium to make up for that which combines with C as it breaks down. The C dose was repeated every 6 hours. She came out of the coma in 24 hours, the only one reported to have done so when bitten as badly (1971).

In another case, a 4-year-old girl bitten by a highland moccasin was seen crying and vomiting a half hour later. She was given 4 grams of C in a vein plus a skin test for antivenin. Before the test was completed the kid was okay, drinking orange juice and wanting to go home. The antivenin was not used. Next day, still slightly feverish, she was given 4 more grams of C and a repeat the following day for good measure. Klenner compared this with a similar bite, judging from fang marks, on a 16-year-old girl who had 3 doses of antivenin but no C. She spent 3 weeks in the hospital and needed morphine to ease the pain.

A few early studies with guinea pigs suggested that C can protect against anaphylactic shock. Others showed no benefit. Klenner appears to have demonstrated its value in humans on a man who suffered a reaction from a puss caterpillar that had crawled across his back, leaving a trail of red welts. The man began to have difficulty breathing, was turning blue when Klenner injected 12 grams of C into a vein. The relief was immediate.

C is a powerful reducing agent and an oxidizer as well. The ability to be either served well when a man in a coma from carbon monoxide poisoning was brought into Klenner's office. Knowing the chemical possibilities, he shot 12 grams of C into a vein. Ten minutes later the man sat up and wondered what had happened.

In treating severe burns Klenner increased the recommended gram or two orally and added intravenous infusion of a half gram for every kilogram of body weight, repeating every 8 hours for several days before lengthening the dose interval to 12 hours. This, along with a 3-percent solution of C used as a topical spray was said to eliminate infection. He wrote: "I have seen eschars 2 inches wide and ½ inch thick, severely infected so that stench had to be controlled with deodorizing sprays, melt away when employing the methods outlined. Ascorbic acid also eliminates pain so that opiates or their equivalent are not required."

It seems that no illness slipped by the doctor without being treated successfully with C. To name a few: pneumonias, diphtheria, encephalitis, hepatitis, mononucleosis, pesticide poisoning, measles, diabetes, tetanus, barbiturate overdose and habitual abortion. He gave C to pregnant women and infants, noting that the only case of quadruple births in southeastern U.S. in which all four survived was managed with this regimen (1971).

He wrote of a case of mononucleosis. The girl had been given last rites and was failing. Her mother, a nurse, asked the doctor to give the girl C. He refused. She gave it herself then, 20 to 30 grams in each unit of intravenous fluid. Recovery commenced and soon the girl walked out of the hospital.

Although it may seem so at the moment, Klenner was not the only physician into high-C therapy prior to 1970. It's just that few took the time to write about it. Abram Hoffer did so. His use of large doses for schizophrenia has already been mentioned. In 1962 W.L. Dalton described a number of viral infections which responded quickly to a commercial preparation containing a large amount of C. The response of patients with infectious mononucleosis, viral pneumonia and hepatitis was termed excellent. His comment on the case of a 20-year-old woman with hepatitis: "It is difficult to comprehend a set of circumstances that would coincidentally explain the marked and rapid improvement in a patient as sick as this girl ... the most dramatic recovery from hepatitis that I have ever observed." He suggested that further investigations be undertaken but of course there was little interest in promoting C for viral therapy. The establishment could recognize the threat to revenue.

E. Greer in 1955 wrote of treating polio cases with 10 grams of C orally taken 4 times a day. His own daughter responded so quickly that he discontinued treatment the next day. The disease then flared up again, prompting a return to the regimen for a week. One patient was given 10 grams of C every 3 hours for 10 days. As did others who used C, he advised that high doses be reduced gradually.

Before-and-after photos by Greer demonstrate the

benefit of high C in preventing the enlargement of the spleen of a patient with polycythemia vera plus leukemia and cirrhosis of the liver. The patient took up to 42 grams a day to keep his spleen from attaining the size of a basketball. It was firm and normal while the intake was high but ballooned out to resemble a lopsided pregnancy whenever the dose was discontinued (1954). Anyone still of the opinion that high C is useless in therapy should look at the pictures if words cannot convince.

Doses needn't always be up in the stratosphere to be of benefit. McCormick wrote of treating scarlet fever with oral and intravenous doses of 2 grams a day. Fever subsided within hours and patients were free of symptoms in 3 or 4 days (1951). A German paper which was summarized in the AMA Journal in 1954 reported that 10 grams of C daily infused for 5 days proved to be an effective treatment for infectious hepatitis.

In 1960 Calleja and Brooks reported a case of hepatitis which had not improved on antibiotics, diuretics, blood transfusions, prednisone and aspiration of excess fluid. Finally the patient was treated successfully with an infusion of 5 grams of C daily. Appetite and well being improved within a week but he was kept on the regimen for 24 days. The physicians were aware of the German report mentioned above but for some reason did not use the 10-gram dose. This may have been the reason for the prolonged recovery. Had they been able to see into the future they would have read Cathcart's 1981 paper that mentioned hepatitis cases being treated successfully with oral doses as high as the bowel permitted.

James Greenwood Jr. in 1964 wrote of treating more than 500 cases of back pain with a half gram of C daily. The patients were advised to increase the dose by 50 to 100 percent if discomfort returned. A number of them were able to avoid surgery just by taking this small amount of C, which is involved in the strengthening of weakened discs. He also found that the percentage of those needing a second operation was reduced. Some stopped taking the extra C after a time and felt the pain returning, a good reminder that the dose should be continuous.

This was Greenwood's experience also. A professor of neurosurgery, he began to recommend C when his own back improved with it. For 10 years his back had bothered, finally getting so bad that after whacking 50 practice golf balls the pain would last for several days. Too many golfing dates had to be cancelled. Originally his dose was 100 milligrams taken 3 times a day. In about 4 months he felt so well that he stopped dosing—but started again when the golf outings were threatened again 3 months later.

Then he told a surgeon friend about his wonderful discovery. To this the surgeon replied that he'd been taking C for his own back problem. Together they settled on the above doses for others having bothersome backs.

In addition to the reports mentioned, the medical literature prior to 1970 contains many more examples which suggest that high-dose C can be helpful in other afflictions. This chapter reports only those results which were achieved clearly by the use of C. Others are questionable. Atkinson's report in 1951 is an interesting observation on Meniere's syndrome but the relationship is not a clear one. He noted that dizziness had been reported in some scurvy cases therefore he dosed a Meniere's patient with high C and other vitamins. The syndrome vanished after 4 years of this treatment. It is worthy of further thought, however, particularly since J. Adam reported in 1939 that Meniere's patients were low-C people and improved when given more of the vitamin.

The case for C in asthma and allergies is a mixed bag in this period yet some good reports appear. The advocacy of high C for the following conditions provide still more food for thought: some skin conditions, bone loss, certain involuntary movements, ileitis and other gut disorders, megaloblastic anemia, cataracts, diabetes and multiple sclerosis. Some of these we'll come back to later.

But scientists kept reminding the healthcare professions that proof of the value of C was lacking except in regard to scurvy. They overlooked a couple of trials, as we'll soon see. They also didn't complain about the lack of financial backing to provide such proof. Not having that support would tend to lock it out of treatment plans.

So all the accounts reported in this chapter so far constitute anecdotal evidence, the sort of experience that doctors historically have relied on to aid in the art of healing. It can be extremely valuable except to those who support the increasing tendency to brush it off as unscientific and therefore worthless. Unless of course common sense intervenes. One must remember that no double-blind controlled scientific trial on humans has ever proved that eating the wrong mushroom can be fatal. Purists don't play scientific hardball in this area. What they see is what they believe, yet it is anecdotal evidence.

Drugs that can help only a few patients are similar to C in that no money can be made from them. For these, the "orphan drug" program was instituted. It allows one company to have exclusive marketing rights to the little-used drug so that the firm won't lose money handling it.

It would seem that society might benefit from a program which considers C as similar to an orphan because it lacks financial backing for scientific trials. The government or a large philanthropic organization wishing to make a substantial contribution to human welfare should fund such trials—carefully supervised to prevent rigging—in order to bring the substance into the mainstream of medical treatment. It might cut the cost of healthcare down a few notches.

The government did fund the following trial via the Army during World War II, as reported in 1947 by D.H. Klasson. He divided 48 men who were sensitive to poison oak into 2 groups of 24 each then pretreated one group with C before exposing both to the oak. The pretreated group was spared the itching while those in the control group exhibited reactions ranging from mild to severe. The amount of C used was surprisingly small—less than a gram daily. Intramuscular injections were tried for treatment of established itches and were seen to shorten the period of discomfort. Doses were repeated every few hours because extra C is cleared from the bloodstream quickly.

Whether such pretreatment would be effective against poison ivy as well as oak is not known. I do know that a continuous intake of a gram daily does not protect against poison ivy, nor does a 16-gram continuous dose. Perhaps a *rise* above the base dose is necessary, as in the treatment of colds and flu. I haven't tried it.

In 1961 McConnell reported the results of an interesting study. He gave 89 patients who'd had from 1 to 4 previous strokes 600 to 800 milligrams of C daily along with bioflavonoids which increase the uptake. During the period of observation only 3 minor strokes occurred in the group. Meanwhile a group of 62 similar patients serving as controls were kept on their usual treatments but not given extra C. This group suffered 12 minor strokes and 18 severe ones, 5 of them fatal. More than half of the patients in each group were below the age of 60, indicating that they were not all oldsters nearing the end of their days.

If the number of patients in each group is equalized, vitamin C is seen to have provided a 14-fold greater protection against recurrent stroke. One would think that by now every stroke-prone individual in the nation would be advised to take at least a gram of C daily. And that other trials would have been conducted to confirm or refute the findings. Nothing shows up in the medical literature.

If C had been a proprietary medicine this protective benefit would have been advertised incessantly for the last 30 years. Many persons would have been helped. Some would still be living. Perhaps in addition to funding for trials, advertising revenue should be provided also.

One would think that a magazine serving the elderly should have followed up on the information about C and strokes when it was brought to the attention of the editors. One would think that they would have looked up the article in the medical literature and reported on the benefit to their readers. This has not been done. Nor has any popular household magazine been interested in passing on the information. All that bull about serving the readers becomes slippery and malodorous when useful information might upset advertisers.

A study reported by Sokoloff in 1966 indicates that C, like most medicines, can help some individuals but not all of them. He gave 60 patients with high cholesterol or heart disease or both an extra amount of C daily—1.5 to 3 grams. No benefit was seen in 10 of them. But in the other 50 the benefits ranged from moderate to impressive.

So it is no cure-all. It is just a good drug which should be kept in mind by all healthcare personnel.

8
The Seventies

Pauling's 1970 book on the common cold awakened public interest in C and turned the attention of scientists to its therapeutic potential and possible toxicity. We've already explored the literature regarding colds and toxicity. This chapter covers other observations and trials of the 1970s but not necessarily in chronological order.

In some ways the medical literature on C in the 70s resembles that of the early 30s. You'll remember that in 1938 Wright characterized it as composed of "truths, errors and debatable questions of which the last mentioned group constitutes the major portion." Debatable questions there were. The colds issue consumed barrels of ink as every group aspiring to be published conducted trials with the same inadequate dosage employed by those who had gone before. One physician allowed that the greatest contribution to the management of a cold is Kleenex. Another pointed out that the public has enough cold remedies and that one more is not needed. Charges of bias and self-interest peppered the letters columns. And the toxicity question was batted back and forth until frazzled.

Whether C could clear out arteries and lower cholesterol levels claimed a bit of space also. In 1972 Spittle cited Sokoloff's 1966 report that extra C helped some patients with heart problems then added her own observations. She had detected a seasonal variation in deaths from heart attack which coincides with the seasonal variation in public consumption of foods containing C. More deaths occurred at the low-intake time of year. In 1973 she reported the results of a double-blind trial on hospital patients given a gram of C daily on admission and for 2 weeks prior to surgery. These patients had about half the number of clots in the deep veins of the legs as were seen in those who were not given extra C. She believed that C could lower cholesterol levels.

In 1977 C.J. Bates reported an 18-month study on 23 relatively healthy oldsters. He found that men with high plasma C levels had more of the "good" cholesterol (HDL). Women did not show the correlation as clearly—probably because they had more favorable HDL levels anyway.

Others reported that extra C had no effect on cholesterol levels. In fact J.D. Davies reported in 1974 that higher C intake actually raised cholesterol levels in nomadic African tribe members whose diet is high in cholesterol. Their cholesterol levels are quite low (135) even though the intake is high, suggesting that life-style or genetic differences may account for the contradictory results.

Spittle's report in 1974 may explain the rise which

was seen in the above investigation. She gave both healthy individuals and those who'd had heart attack extra C an found that the cholesterol count went down in the healthy ones but rose in those with heart disease. She suspected that the reason for the rise is that C begins to clear away excess cholesterol deposits in blood vessels, resulting in higher levels while it is being flushed out. No long-term study to check this theory has been reported.

But extra C was shown to be beneficial during a high-fat meal. We jump ahead to a 1985 report by Bordia and Verma, who studied the blood of healthy males after they had eaten 75 grams of butter. Four hours later the blood platelets had a tendency to clump and cling, not a good thing for blood components to be doing as they flow through the arteries and veins. This tendency could be prevented if the men took a gram of C along with the butter. The researchers also found that 3 grams of C daily decreased clumping and clinging in persons having high levels of blood fats.

A report by C.S. Foster in 1978 points out the perils of going through life with a low level of plasma C. A 24-year-old man with a fungus infection of the cornea had a level in the subclinical scurvy range. He had a history of infections of one sort or another since childhood. Asthma and eczema also. His white blood cells were sluggish, unwilling to do battle. The ulcer of the cornea cleared up in a couple weeks when treated with antifungal agents. Meanwhile the plasma C level rose to high normal in 30 days on 3 grams of C daily. The man's eye condition was followed for 2 years, during which time no more infections occurred.

A 1978 report by Bali and Callaway tells of a man, age 32, who had suffered from migraine headaches for 6 years. To ease the pain he had been taking the drug methysergide (Sansert®) for a year, sometimes with codeine. Interested in other remedies, he found the headaches to be milder and less frequent after several lessons in relaxation techniques.

Then he tried high C while phasing out the other drugs. In 2 months he had quit the drugs entirely in favor of 6 grams of C a day. It is not stated whether the dose was divided, just that whenever he missed taking C in the morning the headaches returned. His physician wondered if a placebo would do as well. A double-blind trial was arranged so that over a 15-day period the man took either capsules of C or a similar-tasting citric-acid placebo. In case a severe headache occurred he was allowed to use his own C to treat it. This he did on 3 days when the headaches were severe.

At the end of the trial period his account of which "medicine" he thought he had taken was compared with the actual substance as determined by its code number. It turned out that he had correctly listed all the days on which he had taken the placebo and those on which he had taken C. As he suspected, he had taken the placebo on the 3 days when the headaches were severe enough to turn him toward his own vitamin C.

Was this a fluke or would high-dose C help a percentage of other individuals suffering from migraine headaches? We'll never know. We should realize by now that no company can make any money by funding a large-scale trial to find out. And unless such a trial shows up in the literature there is not enough evidence to support a statement that C is of value in this area. There may be an interesting connection here with feverfew, a folk medicine which has been used in Europe for centuries. Recently it has become popular as a treatment for migraine, enough so that a British trio headed by J.J. Murphy conducted a randomized double-blind placebo-controlled trial on 59 participants to see if the herb really was effective (1988).

But first the scientists had to grow their own plants because of the quality of purchased preparations. Some of the store-bought stuff had no feverfew at all in the contents. The participants in the trial, not knowing the sequence, took the feverfew for 4 months then the placebo for 4 months—or vice versa—and kept a diary that graded the severity of headaches and other reactions.

Overall, feverfew reduced the number of attacks by 24 percent and significantly lessened the amount of nausea and vomiting. Those with classic migraine were helped the most. They reported a 32 percent reduction in the number of attacks. The active ingredients in feverfew are called sesquiterpene lactones. Vitamin C is a lactone also. Perhaps something about the chemical structure of the two lactones are similar enough to act on some migraine headaches in similar ways.

R.J. Lazarus reported a trial with C in 1970 which

was odd in that the amount of C taken was restricted rather than increased. Scleroderma is a skin condition in which collagen overgrowth plays a role. Collagen, the "glue" protein which holds body connective tissue together, is formed with the aid of vitamin C. Since too much collagen is a feature of scleroderma the reasoning was that less collagen would be formed if less C were present in the diet. But the experimental result didn't mimic the reasoning. The only noticeable effect: one of the patients developed scurvy.

It would seem to be illogical to try high C rather than low C for the above condition and there is no report of such an attempt, probably because many victims of the disease have poor kidneys. To those, high C would be detrimental. It probably would be harmful in cases where kidney function is not affected also.

But the illogic of using high C brings to mind the thinking of early aviators when their flying machines went into a tailspin. They tried every seemingly logical maneuver to keep their machines from augering into the earth without success. Then one day, instead of logically trying to stay away from the earth, a pilot put his plane in a power dive toward it. This broke the spin cycle, allowing him to regain control of the craft.

Would an illogical use of extra C help these patients? Probably not. The blood picture indicates that an autoimmune factor is present. Extra C strengthens the immune system in some ways and to help an immune system which is already attacking body parts is completely illogical.

This applies also in the case of systemic lupus erythematosus, another connective-tissue disorder with an autoimmune factor damaging to body parts. One would not want to stimulate the attacking force to greater activity. Yet lupus patients do not excrete much C in the urine, indicating that the body needs more. More for *what* is the question—for greater body damage by the immune system or for greater body resistance and repair of the damage?

The tendency to form little hemorrhages in the skin is a characteristic of scurvy—and also of lupus. Finkle reported in 1937 that he gave a lupus patient 200 milligrams of C intravenously every day for 6 days then a pint of orange juice daily for more than 2 weeks. Practically no rise in urinary C occurred. The body kept nearly all of it. This excretion pattern was different from the other diseases in the study. The extra C given did not result in any improvement but he didn't report a worsening either.

So what should we make of it? The logic is there for both avoiding and trying high C.

And what should we make of this: In 1972 Poser wrote of a chemist in his mid-thirties whose vision was failing due to lens opacities. Poser had treated patients with high C for years and may have known of a report by Purcell in 1954 stating that people with cataractous lenses have low plasma C; or of a Japanese report in 1956 about C preventing development of cataracts in guinea pigs. So he suggested that the man try 4 grams of C daily for a time. On this regimen the lenses were clear in 4 months. The man was then advised to stop taking the high C dose but he didn't want to. He kept up the regimen for 13 years that the doctor was aware of before he lost contact. The lens of the eye has a relatively high concentration of C, being third highest on the list of body tissues, behind only the pituitary and the adrenals (Hornig, 1976). Currently studies are underway to determine the connection between C and cataracts. How sad that decades go by before studies are undertaken.

Briefly mentioned in the chapter on cancer are the studies on patients with familial polyposis, a condition in which numerous polyps of a precancerous type form in the gut. In 1975 DeCosse reported giving 3 grams of C daily to 5 patients with this condition. Rectal polyps disappeared in 2 of the patients and decreased in size in 2 others. The polyps in one continued to grow, indicating that C had no effect at the dose level used during the time of observation.

Later, in 1982, Bussey, DeCosse and others reported the results of a randomized double-blind placebo-controlled study in which 3 grams of C daily were given to 36 patients. At 9 months into the study they noted a reduction in polyp area in the patients taking C. After 12 months both polyp area and numbers were less in the C group. Later still, in 1988, McKeown-Eyssen reported that only 400 milligrams of C along with an equal amount of vitamin E reduced the number of recurrent polyps in a group under study. The reduction was not as great as when larger doses were used, however. Spigelman in 1990 reported that tissue (leukocyte) C levels were 38 percent higher in persons who did not have polyposis.

Suppose you had identical twins. Suppose you gave one more C for 5 months. Not much more—a half gram daily if they were not extra heavy and between the ages of 6 and 11. If they were older, 11 to 15 years of age, you'd give one an extra 3 quarters of a gram or a full gram, depending on weight. The other twin gets a placebo. Would you be able to notice a difference between them after only 5 months? J.Z. Miller and others (1977) didn't set out to answer that question specifically. Primarily they were investigating the effect of that amount of extra C on cold symptoms but they looked for other developments too. We know by now that such small doses taken continuously have little effect on colds. But some other findings were interesting. Generally, no difference was seen between the twins who were given extra C and their brother or sister whose C intake was only what the diet provided. The greater C intake did not increase thought processes or reaction time. The male twins on the extra amount exhibited better fine muscle control and most had less tremor. The extra-C female twins in the older groups exhibited more tremor, however.

An "entirely unexpected" effect showed up in the young male group, those taking a half gram of C daily. There were 7 pairs of twin boys. In 6 of the 7 pairs, the twin who took extra C grew taller than his brother. In the 5-month period one twin gained an inch in height over his brother. The average gain was slightly more than a half inch. (The twins of the seventh pair matched each other's rate of growth.)

You'd probably notice the difference if one of your twins began to grow taller than the other. Other than that, the effect of extra C in gram amounts or less might be so small as to slip by undetected. At the end of the study the 44 mothers whose twins were in the trial were asked if they could tell which one had taken extra C. Twenty three said they could see no difference. The other 21 said they could—but 4 of them picked the wrong twin. So about 81 percent of those who saw a difference guessed correctly.

The percentage may have been inflated somewhat because 4 of the 44 mothers admitted to having tasted the contents of the different capsules, therefore knew which twin was getting C. The placebo capsule contained starch rather than the usual citric acid which is difficult to differentiate from C by taste. This could have skewed some of the data on colds because the mothers were the ones who judged the severity of cold symptoms. But with such small doses the trial was not a meaningful contest between C and colds anyway.

Sacks and Simpson reported an interesting observation in 1975. A 62-year-old man with Parkinson's disease improved on levodopa, one of the drugs commonly used in treatment. Later he gave it up because of the nausea it caused. He started again on a reduced dose, 3 grams daily, but the amount was barely effective. He was then given extra C in the belief that it might reduce certain side effects. The dose was started at one gram daily and increased to 4 grams as the levodopa intake was cut to 2 grams a day.

In less than a month the man exhibited better head movement and could play the organ again, an ability he had lost several years before. To be sure that the benefit was due to C, a double-blind trial was arranged, using a citric acid placebo instead of C. In less than 2 weeks on the placebo the man reverted to the condition he was in before taking C. When the C dose was resumed he improved again.

The authors suggested that further investigation is needed but there's been no rush to set up a large-scale trial. Recent reports indicate that C is being used in combination with other antioxidants such as vitamin E. This should fuzzy up the results enough so that nothing is positive and the matter will be dropped for another 15 years.

In the fall of 1989 a media blitz promoted the "Parkinson's breakthrough" drug deprenyl, a welcome addition to those used in treating the disease. One of the articles about it stated that further research will include vitamin E. No mention was made of vitamin C, which would work like deprenyl as an antioxidant.

Now why do you suppose vitamin E was picked rather than C? Both are antioxidants but C has been shown to be of value while there is a negative report on E, that of G.M. Stern in 1987. It tells of a horse trainer who showed the first signs of Parkinson's disease at age 56. He began taking levodopa at age 58. Most notable is that for 20 years he had taken at least 400 units of vitamin E every day. Horses seemed to do better on it so he decided to take it too. Clearly, Stern concluded, two decades of vitamin E intake did not prevent the disease or alter the course of it after it came on.

The above account as well as the one on C therapy for the disease appeared in *The Lancet,* a widely read British medical journal. All groups researching Parkinson's surely would be aware of both accounts, thus deepening the mystery as to why vitamin E was favored over C for further testing. Could it be that E is not the great threat to revenue that C is? Or that a research paper featuring E would have a better chance of getting published? Or that E would have a better chance of failure, therefore leading readers to conclude that antioxidants, including C, are of no value in treating Parkinson's? The establishment operates in mysterious ways.

The cause of Parkinson's is unknown but enough is known to generate some interesting thoughts. Ponder this: An epidemic of encephalitis, thought to be of viral origin, occurred worldwide shortly after World War I. In many cases the after effects were identical to those of Parkinson's, which had been described a century before. The two diseases seemed to be separate in name only. One was called postencephalitic parkinsonism because the patient was known to have had encephalitis. When examining the part of the brain affected by both diseases a pathologist could not say which disease caused the damage.

Could a virus be the cause of true Parkinson's disease? It would not be the same one which caused encephalitis first, just as not all cold viruses cause a runny nose first. One wonders if the horse trainer would have contracted Parkinson's if he'd been taking 4 or 5 grams of C daily for 20 years. (That length of time might be necessary. By the time early symptoms are evident about 80 percent of certain brain functions have been lost.)

A number of individuals have been taking 4 to 6 grams of C daily for several years and will continue to do so. No doubt some have a susceptibility to Parkinson's. If one of them ever develops the disease we'll learn that C is no more effective than was vitamin E for the unfortunate horse trainer. As for treating it, maybe some day a group will be given as much C daily as the bowel will tolerate over a period of several years in order to evaluate the effect properly. Maybe even before then the establishment will overcome its pathologic fear of reporting a successful trial and use an adequate dose of C with levodopa or deprenyl for the benefit of those who are ill.

9
The Eighties and Beyond

By 1980 the C-versus-colds issue had ceased to be a major topic in the medical literature. Perhaps that's why Bee in 1980 managed to get a letter published which stated that the trials had not used enough C. He wrote of successfully treating himself and numerous patients with 3 or 4 grams taken up to 6 times a day. But the low-dose trial results of the seventies had already convinced the public that any hope of relief by taking the stuff was just another dream. And those who had taken the low doses—or higher ones improperly—were inclined to agree. Most people, doctors included, had never read Pauling's book and didn't realize that second-hand information had distorted his dose recommendations.

Apparently even the so-called authorities never read Pauling's book—or much of the other medical literature on vitamin C. In 1987 a university diet and nutrition letter, after stating that C hadn't been shown scientifically to prevent or cure colds, added the comment that it wasn't because of a lack of effort to do so. Then the letter went on to say that we are not likely to be deficient in C.

The first comment reflects a quickie scan of cold-trial summaries. The second reflects at best a difference of opinion which can impart a false sense of security. Some authorities are stuck with what they espoused at an earlier date and continue to promote the decrepit line of thought as bolstered by the results of all the inadequate-dose cold trials.

Antonio in *The Merchant of Venice* said the devil can cite scripture for his purpose. Likewise, anyone can cite the medical literature to support a point of view. Advocates of higher C intake really wouldn't go so far as to hint that those who are biased against it are in consort with old speartail, though. A kinder, gentler association, like with retarded pagans, maybe. But well meaning and always true to the faith of the clan in their fashion.

And that faith holds that we are not likely to be deficient in C. An adherent can cite, for example, a 1943 German report showing that smokers do not have lower C levels than nonsmokers while not mentioning a half dozen other studies which show that smokers are indeed deficient in C. The German reference is from Pelletier, whose own report in 1968 confirmed that smokers are deficient, as stated in chapter 1 along with other depleters.

So any statement that we are not likely to be deficient in C should make an exception of smokers. It should also except 95 percent of the institutionalized elderly, 68 percent of elderly out-patients and 20 percent of the "healthy" elderly folk, according to a previously mentioned table which was cited by Cheraskin. His own study of more than 4000 individuals comprised of dental personnel, wives and patients found that substantial percentages of supposedly "normal" groups are deficient in the vitamin. And, as we should realize by now, anyone who is sick is deficient in C if extra amounts are not being taken.

It could be said that from the central issue of colds in the seventies the investigation of C radiated into other areas, suggesting that although the public was snookered on the colds issue the substance still could win a place in modern medicine because of its amazing versatility.

For example: A 58-year-old man who had been diabetic for 13 years developed a persistent infection in his external ear canal. An x-ray showed signs of mastoiditis also—inflammation in the bone behind the ear. Intensive daily care failed to clear up the external infection. Treatment with several antibiotics resulted in only scant improvement. Blood studies then revealed that the white cells exhibited a less than normal rate of movement toward the area where they were needed. To correct the slow response the man was given 3 grams of C daily. Steady improvement followed and in 7 weeks the infection cleared up (Corberand, 1982).

One might suspect that the man's blood level of C had been in the low range where subclinical scurvy can cause all sorts of baffling medical problems. This was not stated. But the choice of C as a last resort indicates that the physicians were aware of its ability to stimulate certain white cells to perform better. And the quantity given indicates that they knew a mere gram of C a day wouldn't suffice.

R. Anderson (1980) tested white cell function in the blood of 5 normal individuals in good health then tested again after they had taken a gram of C daily for a week. The gram dose wasn't enough to turn on the white cells. But 2 grams a day for a week alerted them and 3 grams a day proved better yet. Long ago Nungester and Ames (1948) showed that guinea pig white blood cells start losing their ruggedness and inclination to do battle when the plasma C level drops just a little from the optimum. The sharp drop continues as the C level goes down.

It should astound and anger us if our C level is not checked and brought up to maximum as a first requirement of proper treatment for infections and most other illnesses. It is known that animals which can make their own C internally are programmed by their genetic heritage to keep their blood level of C up to the saturation point. Goldsmith in 1961 and C.W.M. Wilson in 1974 expressed the view that we too would fare better if we did so. We should be reminded of it as often as we're told to drive carefully.

As we've seen, the optimum level for some people may not be attainable by diet alone. Rebora reported in 1980 that certain individuals needed doses of C in the 1- to 2-gram range to achieve remission of recurrent skin infections. And R. Anderson reported in 1981 on 3 children who had a chronic urinary bladder disease along with inactive white blood cells. He kicked the lazy cells with a gram of C daily, which was enough for children, added an antibiotic and resolved the problem.

An adult with a somewhat similar condition, thought to be permanent, was cured after C became a part of the treatment plan. The 48-year-old woman had a history of bladder infections over a 6-year period. This time around the urologists told the woman to take a half gram of C 4 times daily as well as the usual antibiotics. The symptoms disappeared after 6 weeks. Six months later the woman lowered C intake to a half gram a day. The bladder wall was found to be normal 9 months after the start of treatment (Stanton, 1983).

Many papers which report favorable results after the use of extra C have urged that clinical trials be undertaken to explore the percentage of people who might be helped. The findings presented should be all the urging that is necessary but seldom is an expressed or implied urging ever acted upon.

A poignant example is the disregard of even the basic property of C in the management of multiple sclerosis patients. Way back in 1947 Williams and Bullock reported that patients with this disease "improved remarkably well" when given a diet rich in vitamin C. They decided to determine the C status of 9 future cases that came under their care. "All showed a level below normal," they stated. The doctors then made a random check of 11 other hospitalized patients. Only two of those had C levels below normal—a patient with a brain hemorrhage and one with psitticosis (parrot fever, a viral disease which could be expected to draw down C stores). The doctors concluded that multiple sclerosis patients are consistently deficient in vitamin C.

The same year, Williams reported giving a group of multiple sclerosis patients 400 milligrams of C along with 4 glasses of orange juice daily which would bring the total daily intake to a little less than a gram. In 4 months the patients became stronger and had fewer relapses.

The establishment was again reminded of the low C status of multiple sclerosis patients, among others, in a 1954 report by L.J. Cass. A group of them were included in a single-blind study in which 6 were given 4 grams of C daily and 4 were given placebos. After 2 weeks the 6 on C had improved so much that the 4 on placebo were also put on C. Additions brought the total to 12, who were treated in this manner for 4 months with good results.

The disease was severe in 10 of the patients as they'd been hospitalized for over 3 years. Only 3 were able to walk. They all said they felt better on the treatment and all but 2 said they were stronger. Relatives and nurses noticed that the patients could speak better. The author concluded that the observations justified further investigation.

A third reminder of the low C status of these patients came in 1982 from Irwin Stone, a biochemist who had a longtime interest in C. He labeled them a scorbutic group and urged that trials be set up in order to determine the amount of C that should be given. Some time in the next century this may be done. So far, no treatment suggestions for the disease include the administration of extra C.

A good case can be made for moving into high-dose C in the treatment of multiple sclerosis. Considerable evidence exists that points to an infectious agent as the cause of it. Some persons may be carriers of the agent without ever developing the disabilities. An elusive virus may be the culprit—one associated with farm animals, as butchers, leather workers and scientists who studied the brains of sick sheep were seen to have more than their share of the disease. Meat shipped from areas where multiple sclerosis is common has caused outbreaks in areas where it is rare. An autoimmune factor is said to be present but the reports of Cass and Williams indicate that C does not enhance the autoimmune activity.

A suspect in the disease has been detected a few times. In 1982 Melnick reported finding a virus in the spinal fluid of 3 patients with MS and 1 with amyotrophic lateral sclerosis (Lou Gehrig syndrome). Another hint that a virus is involved is that proprietary antiviral drugs relieve fatigue in MS patients (G.A. Rosenberg, 1988).

If so, then high C should be tried. It is a much less toxic antiviral substance and has the added advantage of curing the near-scurvy condition which afflicts these individuals. The 4-gram doses that Cass used are of course far too small for inclusion in a definitive trial. Such a puny amount won't even nick an established cold, a relatively mild viral disease. Researchers should try bowel-tolerance doses or nothing at all so they won't muddy up the results. To date that's been the track record every time C has been investigated in large clinical trials.

Of the practicing physicians who know how to handle C properly, Cathcart, a California physician, has contributed more to the recent medical literature on the subject than anyone, as mentioned earlier. Being a victim of hay fever himself and taking 16 grams of C a day during moderate exposure to the allergens, he knows that C intake must be increased to the bowel-tolerance limit during greater exposure.

A few patients will see no dramatic decrease in symptoms until the bowel-tolerance limit is reached. Lower doses may not produce much benefit at all. It appears that a threshold must be reached, at which point C becomes quite effective (1985). As mentioned earlier, he found that about 80 percent of his patients could take oral doses in this manner without experiencing any nuisance side effects. He believes that some side effects such as mouth sores or light rashes may be due to residual chemicals used in manufacture of the substance. Changing source of supply or trying calcium ascorbate or sodium ascorbate rather than the acid form may eliminate the problem.

The initial diarrhea that some individuals experience often disappears after a few days as the gut adjusts so that larger maintenance doses may be taken. Sometimes the oral doses are tolerated better after therapy is commended intravenously. As opposed to a maintenance dose, an acute diseased condition is different, usually allowing a tremendous amount of C to be taken daily in doses an hour or less apart. Cathcart believes that any acute viral disease can be subdued quickly with massive doses of C but the entrenched, chronic viral conditions may not be routed completely although symptoms are lessened.

As did Klenner, Cathcart draws on a large store of clinical experience for examples of the versatility of high-dose C. The wide range of beneficial applications is thought to be due to "some common pathologic processes" which are rendered harmless by the antioxidant and free-radical scavenging action of the large doses.

In his earlier years when he did orthopedic surgery he found that much of the confusion elderly patients exhibited after hip replacement could be prevented with high C. To block asthma attacks induced by exercise, massive doses taken before, during and after the exertion are recommended (1986). The dose of course varies with the individual and must be determined by experimenting.

As McCormick had reported in 1951, Cathcart also saw the rash and high temperature of scarlet fever vanish in a few hours when patients were given large amounts of C. Another type of rash, that from penicillin given elsewhere, disappeared in a few minutes after intravenous C. He noticed that C enhances the effect of antibiotics, as has been reported by others and that food poisoning may be subdued when high C is taken. Oddly, the diarrhea seen in these cases is diminished rather than increased by the high dose.

The patient with confusing allergies has received

considerable attention in high C therapy. If the dose is kept high enough for a time an allergist may use C as an aid to diagnosis by shortening the reactions to chemicals so that the offending ones can be spotted quicker.

It is evident that his success with C in allergies is due to long experience plus an understanding of how certain allergies come about. The inflamed gut, from yeast, ameba or other parasites allows larger food particles to be absorbed than should be. The body doesn't like this. Reactions follow. High C reduces the inflammation so the gut can function better. Clearing out the parasites with appropriate drugs is of course part of the treatment.

In 1984 Cathcart published a paper on the treatment of AIDS with doses of vitamin C ranging from 50 to over 200 grams a day. For maximum absorption before diarrhea is triggered the dose may be divided and given hourly. Proper use will suppress the symptoms and bring the patient out of the near-scurvy condition which accentuates the profound weariness. Good results depend on keeping the dose as high as possible after clearing out the gut parasites that are present in most male homosexuals.

Parasites add to the burden on the immune system. Some AIDS symptoms may flare up during the process of eliminating the parasites, causing patients to think that C is of no value. Yeast infection (Candida) is also a problem. Taking less sugar and refined carbohydrates along with ingesting more foods having lactobacillus cultures tend to prevent reinfection. The high C dose recommended is a mixture of 3 parts ascorbic acid and 1 part calcium-magnesium-potassium ascorbate. The acidic substance should not be allowed to linger in the mouth because it can etch tooth enamel over a period of time.

Increased food sensitivities seen in AIDS patients add still another problem so that offending foods and even the wrong brand of C must be eliminated. Ascorbate made from the sago palm starch or cassava root (tapioca) rather than corn starch is sometimes better tolerated, probably because the residuals of different chemicals used in synthesis are not as bothersome to some individuals.

Cathcart's experience plus that of other physicians treating AIDS with C may account for the increased longevity seen in the group. He believes that the full-blown disease can be prevented if all those who have been exposed to the virus would take as much C as the bowel will tolerate every day for life. He wonders if a complete cure is possible if, in the early stage, a continuous infusion of high C amounting to 180 grams or more a day were to be given for a long period.

In 1987 Pauling and Cameron presented to the President's Commission on AIDS a statement to the effect that large doses of C merit consideration in the therapeutic approach to the disease. Included were 6 personal accounts by individuals who'd had the full-blown disease and had gone to the Pauling Institute in Palo Alto to tell of their experience. All had either quit standard treatment schedules or decided against the therapy. The most effective element in self treatment was dosing with 15 to 20 grams of C a day.

Four of the 6 appeared to be in excellent health. One
looked well but his immune system continued to be
substandard. The sixth man still had the typical skin
lesions but the nurse who came with him said they
were slowly disappearing. Pauling asked for support
of a research program to see whether the anecdotal
evidence presented would lead to an accepted
method of treating AIDS. The Pauling Institute, a
nonprofit organization dependent on private dona-
tions, needed financial help to conduct a controlled
trial which would test C against proprietary antivi-
rals and a placebo.

In spite of the evidence gathered over the last 50
years that C is an antiviral substance the request for
funding was turned down. Perhaps the pharmaceutical industry has truly succeeded in erasing the antiviral record from official memory. Or perhaps the
Commission members based their decision on the
results of the cold and cancer trials in the assumption
that they accurately reflected what could be expected
from an AIDS trial. Having absolutely no experience
with high-dose C may have been a factor also. Plus
fear of panic in the establishment at the thought of a
successful trial with C. Or the thought of having to
share access to the billions up for grabs to develop
more expensive drugs.

The Pauling Institute abandoned hope for a human
trial but did do less expensive studies in test tubes,
using C in amounts that can be supplied to body
tissues. The scientists found that C suppressed
growth of the AIDS virus in cells without interfering
with the activity of the cell itself. C was seen to act

in a different manner than does AZT, leading to a suggestion that combined treatments would be more effective (Harakeh, 1990). How long will it be before this is mentioned in the news? Valsecchi stated in 1984 that workers in more than 50 occupations risk exposure to chromium salts. He reported the problems of a 52-year-old radiologist whose hands were sensitive to the chromates in a processing solution. Barrier creams were of no value and gloves were a hindrance so he endured the discomfort and spent the weekends treating his hands. He then tried an ointment of 10-percent C, applied 3 times a day. The hands slowly began to improve. In 2 months the dermatitis had vanished.

It was not stated whether the man's plasma C level had been determined. One wonders if the sensitivity would occur in an individual having a high level of C. The question can be asked in any number of therapies. For example, J.V. Wright reported in 1984 that the nausea and vomiting of pregnancy can be relieved with 25 milligrams of C along with certain other vitamins. That small amount suggests that maybe the placebo effect did more than the vitamins. Maybe not, however, when one considers that pregnancy depletes the body of C. Would the nausea have occurred at all if the plasma C level had been determined and kept high as a routine part of the management of the pregnancy case? Or in the management of *any* illness?

In 1984 Bober wrote that of 255 consecutive referrals to a psychogeriatric assessment unit, 75 percent had blood levels low in C or folate or both. Would

they have needed referral to the unit if those levels
had been maintained at high normal as they grew
older? Another question: why don't all units checking on the health of oldsters test for C level? They
test for folate and B-12 but not C. The blind spot
seems to be as opaque as ever.

And not only in the areas concerned with the elderly. Commercial formulas for babies try to imitate
human milk as closely as possible—except for C content. Byerly reported in 1985 that human milk contains *twice* the amount of C that is recommended for
infant formulas. Nature wants babies to be given
adequate C. Salmenpera reported in 1984 that exclu-
sively breast-fed babies have plasma C levels which
are usually above that seen in babies on formula,
never below. The plasma C in breast feeders was
found to be about twice as high as that in their mothers, indicating that high levels of the substance are
vital to the health of babies. The mother's plasma C
reaches a low about 2 months after the baby is born
when no supplement is taken.

Treatment with the hormone ACTH tends to depress some patients, according to Cocchi (1980). He
reported using intravenous doses of C to bring patients, ages 5, 7, 19, and 29 out of the mental state
with intravenous doses of C. Investigators have
looked at C in the treatment of mental illness for
years and occasionally interesting reports are published. In 1984 Kay reported the results of a double-
blind trial which compared C and the chelating substance EDTA with the antidepressant drug amitrip-
tyline. Both treatments worked equally well on de-

pressed patients but manic patients responded better to lithium than to C and EDTA. Studies have shown that people who are subject to manic-depressive mood swings have higher than normal amounts of vanadium in the tissues. prompting the thought that it could be a factor in the disease. This was the reason for using EDTA. It hooks onto the vanadium in order to remove the excess.

After the presentation by Heikkila of a paper on certain brain chemistry at the Third Conference on Vitamin C (published in 1987) the discussion turned to its value in megadoses and whether they have any effect on the body. The answer is emerging, a scientist replied, megadoses may actually override some systems. So, the questioner mused, Pauling just may have a point about C and mental illness.

As for what megadoses can do for the body in other illnesses, it should be obvious by now. But how large doses accomplish the job is not known for sure. Cathcart's 1985 paper notes that the substance is an antioxidant and free-radical scavenger. His 1991 paper treats the subject at length. A radical is a molecule which has lost an electron. It becomes a free radical when it breaks out of the normal scheme of things. Compare it to a misplaced plant, which becomes a weed when it's in the garden. Like weeds, free radicals are a burden. They've lost an electron and want it back and will rob to get it. An unruly mob of them damages tissue, generates more of their kind and starts a domino effect.

The body has systems that halt the process but illness signifies that the systems are overwhelmed, that the bacteria or viruses are producing free radicals faster than the systems can zap them. The chemistry of this high-speed electron pinball game is the core of Cathcart's paper. Massive doses of C saturate the tissues with jillions of extra electrons so that the body systems are not totally removed from their normal "housekeeping" duties by the push-and-shove of electron upmanship.

Spare electrons are everywhere because C has supplied them. It is not the vitamin duty that C is into here. It is the scavenging of free radicals due to the unique structure of the C molecule which allows it to deliver high-energy electrons. C is not the best molecule available but appears to be better suited for the job than others.

Cathcart stated that if a cheaper and better tolerated substance than C could be found he would use it instead. The body doesn't need high C for its vitamin activity. It needs the electrons that can be ripped off easily from each molecule of C. As he put it, diseases involving free radicals can be ameliorated by the electrons carried by C when used properly in large doses. He concludes: "The ultimate use of ascorbate in massive doses is inevitable . . ."

Meanwhile we can still round up reports on the benefits of C doing duty as a vitamin. E.J. Caldwell noted in 1988 that a low blood level of C is associated with problems during pregnancy. One wonders how long such information will continue to be published before everyone gets the message.

The message is slow to circulate in other areas as well. Klenner in 1971 stated that for 17 years he had observed the effect of daily intake of 10 grams of C by diabetics. He found that 60 percent of them could be controlled by diet and that amount of C. The other 40 percent needed insulin but less of it.

J.A. Vinson reported on the benefit seen when 2 grams of C daily were taken by 8 diabetics for 3 weeks (1989). The sorbitol buildup in red blood cells decreased by over 44 percent. An earlier trial with 4 individuals resulted in a 56 percent reduction. Sorbitol is suspected of being a cause of diabetic complications. The author suggests that a little extra intake of C might provide a simple means of preventing or lessening the complications of diabetes without the use of drugs.

Don't get out your stopwatch to see how long before this information is conveyed to diabetics via the establishment.

B.D. Cox reported a study on 12 diabetics who were given a gram of C daily for 2 months in order to assess changes in capillary fragility in the skin and the eye retina. The diabetics were also given a placebo for a month, either before or after the time on C so that the effect of just taking pills would not be a factor. During the time they were taking C the diabetics had stronger capillaries, coming close to matching those of the nondiabetics tested.

No change was seen in the retina during the time on extra C but afterward one of the diabetics had a series of small retinal hemorrhages. It was suggested that they were due to the sudden withdrawal of the extra C (1975). Here is one more indication that systemic conditioning occurs, even at lower doses. Percentagewise, the drop from a gram a day to what the normal diet provides is tremendous. Those who are young and healthy probably wouldn't notice but in a diabetic or the sick or elderly the drop might trigger problems.

Another indication that systemic conditioning occurs at lower doses is seen in a report by L. Martin in 1974. A man who had been taking a gram of C daily for 2 years was told to stop. Four days after discontinuing the dose his urinary excretion of C had dropped to nearly zero—one fifth of a milligram a day. Normal is about 40 milligrams a day. If the body hadn't been conditioned to processing the extra C his urinary excretion would have dropped just to normal from the higher output that a gram a day generates.

10
Odds and Ends

Humans and other primates lack just the final enzyme in the sequence which the liver uses to convert glucose to vitamin C. It is said to have been lost 60 million years ago. Was it lost completely? Scientists have studied C for less than a hundred of those 60 million years. It is an intriguing thought that somewhere among the billions of people on earth are a few who can make their own vitamin C internally. If such talent can be found in a few guinea pigs then humans might still have it also.

As do humans, guinea pigs exhibit considerable variability in resistance to scurvy when C is eliminated from their diet. Odumosu found a few female guinea pigs that did very well on a no-C diet (1973). Ginter (1976) stated that of the thousands of guinea pigs studied in his laboratory over a period of 20 years, a very small number were able to make C internally, probably less than one in a thousand.

Typically, a guinea pig on a no-C diet will show signs of scurvy between day 17 and day 23 and would die on or about day 28. Ginter found 2 male animals that showed no sign of C deficiency while on a no-C diet for 4 months. Two years later he again noticed that a male guinea pig continued to excrete large amounts of C 4 months after being put on a no-C diet. The little fellow was kept on the diet for 33 weeks, thriving all the while. It weighed over 2 pounds when it died, apparently of pneumonia. At autopsy the amount of C in its liver was twice that which is normally found in guinea pigs receiving 10 milligrams of C a day.

Would there by one human in, say, a million who has the ability to make C internally? If such there be, for him or her is reserved a day in the sun. More publicity than winning a lottery—maybe as much money, too. This enterprising society should offer a finder's fee and initiate a search.

For years many authorities claimed that C had no value beyond its nutritive effect as a vitamin. Today it is recognized that in higher doses C acts as a drug. Drug and nutrition properties are determined in part by the way a molecule is built. Like many chemicals, ascorbic acid has an isomer—a twin but not an identical twin. One atom is hooked a bit differently. Vitamin C is L-ascorbic acid. Its twin is D-isoascorbic acid, also called erythorbic acid. The D substance, not found in nature, is practically useless as a vitamin. From 20 to 40 times more of it is needed to equal the protection against scurvy that ascorbic acid provides. Yet it does exhibit some of the enzyme activity of C.

So what could we expect from D-isoascorbic acid in a battle against the common cold? To find out, Clegg and Macdonald set up a double-blind trial in which one group of people took a gram of real vitamin C daily, a second group took a placebo and a third group took a gram of useless D-isoascorbic acid, for 15 weeks (1975). The results of the trial confirmed that a gram of C a day, like a placebo, is of little value in treating colds. But what a surprise— the group taking D-isoascorbic acid logged 34 percent fewer colds than those on placebo and about 32 percent fewer than those on C. Blood studies done during the trial found that D-isoascorbic acid caused no change in body functions, therefore is as harmless as C itself at that dose level.

If a gram of the D substance is so great as a cold remedy how much more effective would 5 or 6 grams be? We don't know because no further trials have been reported. This shouldn't surprise us. The financial disadvantage of exploring the benefits of the D substance is also a twin to that of the L substance.

The D substance is widely used in food processing—in hot dogs as sodium erythorbate, for example. In 1989 Sauberlich estimated that more than 200 milligrams of erythorbic acid per capita goes into our food every day. This could be a health problem indirectly because erythorbate registers as vitamin C on urine and blood tests, making them worthless. Fasting must now be longer—overnight—or a false reading would result. The body would seem to be well supplied with C when in fact it might be needing much more.

Klenner in 1971 stated that his family survived the flu epidemic of 1918 "when scores about us were dying" because the Klenners drank a bitter tea brewed from the plant called boneset (Eupatorium perfoliatum). The powdered leaf and flower of the plant have been used in folk medicine since colonial times. Also called Indian sage, boneset was listed in the U.S. Pharmacopeia from 1820 to 1916 and in the National Formulary from 1926 to 1950, according to V.J. Vogel in *American Indian Medicine* (1970, University of Oklahoma Press, Norman).

The name boneset is said to have sprung from the use of the tea to treat breakbone fever, a common name for dengue, which is caused by a mosquito-borne virus. The assumption may be wrong, however. Merriam Webster's Ninth New Collegiate Dictionary indicates that the word boneset was in use in 1764 while breakbone fever came into use almost a hundred years later, around 1860. The fever may have been named to fit the cure rather than vice versa.

Whatever, Klenner had the plant analyzed for C content then calculated that his boyhood dosings of boneset tea provided him with 10 to 30 grams of C at one time. He must have sipped a bucket or two of concentrated brew. Using a reasonably accurate test strip made by Merck's German unit, I found that a tea made from 4 big boneset leaves contained over 200 milligrams of C. Tea from the dried flowers yielded only about a fourth as much and the same drink made from the roots, said to be of value, contained very little C.

No other common non-garden plant tested approached boneset leaves in C content. It appears that the Indians knew what they were doing when they used it for various ills. As for certain other advocated remedies, let's just say that they had also discovered the placebo effect.

Green needles of the red pine tree proved to be equal to boneset in C content. The brown needles of the previous year's growth, being drier, contained twice the C per unit of weight. Tea made from the same weight of green white-cedar sprigs, the arborvitae which is said to have cured Cartier's men, contained about 100 milligrams of C.

In the search for high C in plant parts or fruit, the list of contenders probably started with lemons and oranges then moved to garden peppers, which contain about twice the C as an equal weight of oranges. Nutrition manuals indicate that the bell pepper supplies about 1.3 milligrams of C per gram of pulp. Topping that are the guava and black currant with about 1.7 milligrams of C per gram. Some guavas test higher—3 milligrams per gram—according to Asenjo (1946). Further concentration is found in the fruit of the baobab tree, which can range over 4 milligrams (W.R. Carr, 1955); and the fruit of the tropical tree *Phylanthus emblica* with 8 milligrams of C per gram of pulp (Asenjo).

Those figures are minor league compared to rose hips and the acerola, however. G. Hunter reported in 1943 that the Russians had found rose hips to be a good source of C. He and Tuba collected hips from 3 varieties growing around Edmonton, Alberta.

Hips just covered with water, boiled 15 minutes and mashed yielded 20 milligrams of C per teaspoon of filtered fluid, yet most of the C was still in the pulp. The higher the latitude the greater the concentration of C, they observed. This may be why rose hips in Alberta averaged more than 47 milligrams per gram while Asenjo in Puerto Rico found them yielding 17 milligrams per gram.

His investigation of the West Indian cherry led to its being named the richest natural edible fruit source of C. Also called Barbados cherry or acerola, the fruit looks somewhat like a standard cherry but is not related to it. Asenjo found that juice from the unripened fruit contains about 30 milligrams of C per gram. When red ripe the C content is somewhat lower. Current nutrition manuals rate each gram of acerola, pulp or juice, at 16 milligrams of C.

In 1956 Clein reported that acerola juice caused no reaction in sensitivity tests given to 100 children, half of whom were the allergic type. Eight of the hundred had reactions to orange juice, indicating that acerola can be substituted when orange juice can't be taken yet something completely natural is desired.

Recent additions to the array of cold and flu medicines are the hot-toddy types. You pour powder from a packet into a cup of hot water and, if the TV ads are nonfiction, relief is seen to arrive before the commercial ends. A look at the list of active ingredients on the packet suggests that the mix is an attempt to be all things to all people. It may be shotgun therapy's finest hour.

A look at the inactive ingredients generates a surprise; some brands contain ascorbic acid. How much ascorbic acid is a secret. The pharmacist couldn't tell me. He said that manufacturers are not required to reveal the amount of inactive ingredients in a product. The assumption is that ascorbic acid is an inactive ingredient, a hint that not much went into the formula. But how much?

I bought a box in order to satisfy my curiosity. The reasonably accurate test strip showed that a packet contained 100 milligrams of ascorbic acid. Taking the limit of 4 packets a day would provide the cold sufferer with 400 milligrams of C. Every little bit helps, even if only for duty as a vitamin. But for much less money one could take a gram an hour of ascorbic acid alone and be more apt to experience real relief.

To linger on the subject, a recent television news segment featured a professor with a group of people playing cards during an experiment to determine how the cold virus is spread. At the end of the interview the reporter asked the professor what he does when he comes down with a cold. The professor replied that he never gets a cold—he takes a couple grams of vitamin C. Now why do the lyrics of a song come to mind—about the daisies in the dell that seem to know but they don't tell. Those in academe seem to know but, scientifically, they don't tell that C is an effective treatment for colds.

These facts are known: our immune system deteriorates as we age. Cancer, cataract, stroke, heart attack, diverticulitis, fatigue and a number of other afflictions without end become more prevalent as we grow older. Also known: our plasma C level declines steadily as the years go by. Scientists cannot be so bold as to assert that a connection exists but the results of their studies surely suggest it. We've been alerted to the possibility in previous chapters. A second look is appropriate.

Consider cataracts. Varma and Richards suggested in 1988 that C may bolster certain protective mechanisms in the eye that slow down as we age, that "sluggish transport" of C into the eye may lead to the formation of some cataracts. They point out that vital parts of the eyes of daytime animals contain more C than those of nocturnal species. For what reason? Perhaps this: the free radicals which are generated by light as it passes through the eye are of course more numerous in daytime animals. More C is needed by the daytime eye in order to reduce them. The unanswered question is how much more C intake is needed to overcome the sluggish transport problem in order to be preventive.

Another question: does the decline in both tissue C and the immune system allow Paget's disease of the bone to develop? It is a disease of middle age and beyond. One can readily suspect that here is another of those maladies in which a virus plays a part. Around our bones we have bone-building cells and bone-removal cells. Normally they are supervised by a biological foreman of some sort so that all goes well. In Paget's disease of the bone the dismantling and rebuilding takes place at random, causing thickened, bowed or weakened bones, sometimes accompanied by pain.

The virus suspicion is reinforced by the sighting of foreign particles in the bone-removal cells. Electron microscope pictures suggest that the material belongs to a virus. Other detection techniques have implicated a virus of the measles group but less common groups haven't been ruled out.

In 1978 Basu reported a trial in which 16 victims of the disease took 3 grams of C daily to see if it would ease the pain. The dose was taken for only 2 weeks and no placebo group was used to compare treatment "medicines." Nevertheless, the results were encouraging. Pain vanished completely in 3 of the 16 and partially in another 5. The other 8 were not helped by that small dose.

The disease afflicts fewer than one in a hundred in the U.S. therefore the susceptibility to it is rather low, as is the priority to conduct further trials using massive doses of C for months. When this is done we'll know whether high C can not only relieve pain but inhibit the virus and halt the random destruction.

Alzheimer's is one of the most feared of the age-related problems that are being studied intensely at present. Two similar diseases, Creutzfeldt-Jakob and kuru are of viral origin but there is no good reason to suspect that a virus is involved in Alzheimer's. If it should turn out to be so, the virus will be one of the most elusive yet. That which causes kuru, the brain disease of ritual cannibalism, is elusive enough. Its incubation period in humans may extend beyond

30 years. A virus operating on an even longer time schedule is not an impossibility. Nor is just a viral particle.

We shouldn't expect to see any reports of trials using high C to determine whether it would be useful in treating Alzheimer's but animal studies to observe its effect on amyloid deposits have been conducted. Amyloid is a sort of sludge protein which is found in the brain tissues of both Creutzfeldt-Jakob and Alzheimer's patients. It is not limited to just these diseases, however.

Baltz reported in 1984 that C has no effect on amyloid deposits but Ravid found that C could clear them out in mice (1985). Baltz reported in 1987 that mice having amyloid lived considerably longer when taking extra C. She suggested that humans probably would also.

One could argue that an Alzheimer's patient has nothing to lose by starting a daily 15- to 20-gram C regimen because even some of the rare side effects could be no worse. It is depressing to have to grasp at straws because the potential of high-dose C has not been explored fully. We'll know much more than we do now if someone who has been taking 15 grams of C daily for years should become a victim of Alzheimer's. Only then can we be sure that high C has no value in treating it.

Those shocking descriptions of sailors sprawled on deck exhausted, teeth falling out, old scars opening up and blood oozing from purple pools in the skin are horrors of the past that are not seen today. Only the early stages of scurvy are written up from time to time. The disease doesn't always follow a set pattern and may afflict the sexes somewhat differently. Although fatigue is a constant, gum trouble is not always seen. Little bleeding areas of the skin, starting with a small dot due to capillary breakdown is also seen in all cases. They enlarge and unite into splotches.

Anne Walker described 7 cases of adult scurvy in women in 1967. The main features were mental depression and edematous "woody" swelling of the legs with bleeding from purple splotches on the calves, less so from a network of potential bleeding sites along the shins, which were tender. (The tendency to bleed is greater in the legs because fluid pressure is greater there when one is standing or sitting.) Of interest is that the depression cleared a few days after therapy with C was started, suggesting that the depression of scurvy differs from the usual types.

A classic sign of scurvy was present in 3 of Walker's patients: a condition called follicular keratosis in which the hairs of the skin are surrounded by a horny substance, causing skin roughness. Each follicle may have a red ring of inflammation around it and the hairs themselves may be coiled or "swan-necked."

In 1985 J.B. Reuler wrote of 3 scurvy cases in men, ages 39, 55 and 61. Again, the common feature was swelling and tenderness of the legs, purple splotches and tendency to bleed. Rough skin was also present and sore gums bothered the two who had teeth.

Reuler stated that 75 percent of scurvy patients are anemic because of no C in the diet to enhance iron absorption and not enough C in the tissues to promote iron utilization. R.E. Hodges in 1969 and 1971 and R.E. Baker in 1969 reported on the scurvy picture seen when volunteers were put on a no–C diet. Only one of a 5-man group developed swollen legs. This occurred long after other signs had appeared. Fatigue, shoulder and leg aches and red spots in the skin appeared first, 3 and 4 weeks into the experiment. Rough skin, coiled hairs and gum trouble came about the sixth week. One man dropped into depression which increased the drain of his C reserve.

In Sauberlich's 1989 report on women volunteers taking a no–C diet no mention is made of leg swelling. Six of the 11 women showed signs of scurvy by day 24 with gum trouble. Nine developed acne. One had aching knees on day 22 and red spots by day 25. Because the experiment was short the disease did not progress to more serious problems. One woman needed 90 milligrams of C daily to recover from the gum trouble. Compare this with the following paragraph.

A man in Hodges' study recovered from all the afflictions of rather severe scurvy while taking only 6.5 milligrams of C a day (from *Nutrition Reviews,* Jan. 1986). He had fatigue and lassitude, gum trouble, enlarged saliva glands, dry eyes and mouth, rough skin, coiled hairs, bleeding red spots, joint swelling and pain, bleeding into nerve sheaths which impaired leg function, labored breathing and 21 pounds of water retention resulting in edema of the legs and elsewhere. He spent 91 days on the no-C diet and 123 days on the slow-recovery dose. What a way to get out of work.

The interaction between copper and extra C in both the gut and bloodstream is a small cloud on the horizon that has been pointed out by some researchers. It may loom larger when more people begin taking 5 to 20 grams of C a day for long periods. E. B. Finley reported in 1983 that a half gram of C daily for 64 days was antagonistic to copper status in young men. R. A. Jacob reported in 1987 that 605 milligrams of C taken daily for 3 weeks dropped copper activity by 21 percent. At these low doses, however, it didn't seem to matter. People have been taking much larger doses for years without noticing any ill effects. But because of individual differences and increasing use of much higher doses, we may see a problem turn up eventually.

When high C and copper are in the gut at the same time, less copper is absorbed. Eventually the body could become depleted. What happens then? Heart trouble. In 1980 Klevay reported that a man on a copper-depletion diet for 105 days developed irregular heartbeats and a 16-percent rise in cholesterol. Earlier (1975), Klevay presented some interesting data to support a belief that a high body ratio of zinc to copper is a factor in coronary heart disease.

Perhaps high-C dosers should not take C and mineral supplements containing copper at the same meal.

11
On High C

Scientific reports in the literature tell us very little about dose regimens using C in amounts greater than 10 grams a day. Usually the double-blind placebo-controlled trials have employed doses in the range of 5 grams or below. Scientists with expertise in the low doses therefore have limited knowledge about the effect of higher doses. *"Here be dragons"* is in effect all they can write, as did the early mapmaker in the empty expanse representing unexplored areas.

What we know of very high dosing comes from the anecdotal reports of practicing physicians intent on helping sick patients. Their observations of the sick for long periods may be of greater value than a one-month scientific trial on healthy subjects reported by a doctoral candidate whose expertise peaks briefly in one area before C is abandoned in favor of other pursuits. The quick study may leave something to be desired in the way of accuracy, too.

I participated in a study by a doctoral candidate in which a group of us swallowed some radioactive liquid then exhaled into an apparatus until the condensate of our breath moisture filled a small vial. Much fuss was made about making sure our exhalations went into the gadgetry, not into open air. ... The noon hour was approaching. An assistant in the study had to eat on time then hurry to another activity. But at high noon one fellow's condensate had filled only two thirds of the vial. No matter. He was disconnected and the vial filled with some of the ice water used in the process. Other vials may have been topped off in the same manner.

The results of such a "scientific" determination would be as meaningless as a report by a guy who had a dozen different drinks then picked the one that took him out. Speaking of alcohol brings to mind the treatment in the news of a report by Susick on the effects of 5 grams of C daily taken for 2 weeks prior to ethanol consumption (1987). The findings were condensed to a short statement that extra C clears alcohol from the blood 10 percent faster than normal. No mention of less fatty junk in the liver or other benefits. Or that one fourth of the people in the study actually cleared alcohol *slower* after taking C. One individual cleared it 15 percent slower than his rate before taking C.

Picture what that could lead to: A 15-percent-slower type doses on high C then freeloads 10 percent more booze at a convention, expecting to rise next morning with only the usual blahs. Instead, he's drummed into consciousness with nerves so raw that he hears the surf of both oceans and the spider rapelling down the drapery sounds like a battleship dropping anchor.

Never trust your future to statements in a news item.

What motivates a reasonably healthy individual to try dosing with C above the 10-gram range? Klenner took from 10 to 20 grams a day but made no mention of specific benefits. Pauling once wrote of taking 3 grams a day. Later his dose was reported to be up to 10 grams. His most recent book, *How To Live Longer And Feel Better* (W.H. Freeman & Co., New York, 1986), puts the daily dose at 18 grams, plus more at the onset of weariness or a cold. From this he derives an "increased feeling of well being."

Cathcart named a specific problem, hay fever, which is countered with 16 grams or more daily. Sherry Lewin, a scientist mentioned earlier, credited a gram a day with banishing symptoms which had preceded an earlier heart attack. Increasing to 2 or 3 grams daily provided relief from cold sores and dosing with up to a gram an hour suppressed colds. I met a man, about 40 years old, who takes 36 grams a day. This is his bowel-tolerance limit when he is not ill. When asked why he took so much he said that he is subject to infections if he doesn't. He is a scientist who does know something about the effects of very high doses of C.

There must be hundreds of people who are taking from 10 to 20 grams daily. Their experiences would be of considerable value if the establishment were inclined to listen. Someone was so inclined several years ago. Readers of a professional journal were asked to send such anecdotal evidence to an address in Texas. No collection has been published in the medical literature, however.

My own experience should expand the meager information in this area. I had been taking a half gram of C daily for years in a multivitamin tablet. At about age 60 I increased the intake to a gram daily by adding a half-gram tablet of C only. My interest in the vitamin was increasing and I wanted to see if the doubled dose would produce any noticeable difference. It didn't. Colds and flu continued to occur at the same rate and my quota of a half dozen cold sores a year remained undiminished. I did not try higher doses, trusting that the scientific trial results with respect to colds were meaningful and the warnings of side effects should be heeded.

Aging doesn't seem to be a gradual process. Instead, we seem to drop down periodically from a series of plateaus. One day we discover ourselves on a lower one, in a decreased state of well being. The drop during the year after I turned 68 was quite noticeable. Still I was in good health, had no habits damaging to it and made enough physical work for myself to call it exercise. But that year a neck muscle developed an uncomfortable crick which lasted all summer. Every earth-moving session with the wheelbarrow haunted me with pain in the lower back for days afterward.

I had always been a favorite growth medium for fungus. Any laxity in powdering my toes resulted in a flare-up of athlete's foot. Now the little toenail began to thicken and a dry type of fungal expedition started advancing across the top of my left foot just behind the toes. Then a moist itchy area inside the left ear added another theater of action. About every fourth day I swabbed the spot with antifungal cream, sometimes switching to iodine to give the enemy a change of harassment.

In March 1986 at age 69 I abruptly raised my C intake to 6 grams a day, taken in 4 divided doses after meals and bedtime snack. At first I used tablets but soon switched to powder dissolved in water. To dull the acidity I mixed in various juices before settling on a quarter of a cup of apricot nectar. It worked well as a mask for both the acid form and the bitter calcium ascorbate. Eventually I went back to using water because the tartness and bitterness ceased to bother. (About a third of my dose is calcium ascorbate.)

I was fortunate in not getting the idea to make up a solution that would last all day. Later, on reading Sherry Lewin's book, I learned that half of the C in a cup of tap water is destroyed if the solution is left standing for a few hours. This is due to the air in water plus traces of iron and copper. Copper readily destroys C. Lewin also advised that some tablets can lose up to 80 percent of their potency if left at room temperature for a year. For storage, a cool dry place is recommended. The refrigerator is not a good place to keep the supply that is to be used daily. When the container is taken out and opened regularly the cold contents attract moisture and in time will become lumpy if the C is in powder form or soggy if in tablet form.

The first noticeable benefit from the 6-gram regimen showed up within a week. The ear didn't demand to be swabbed to quell the itch as it should have. Next to vanish were the neck crick and the low-back pain. Slower to resolve were the athlete's foot, the fungal advance atop the foot and the thickened toenail. But even now at higher doses the toenail still shows signs of fungal activity.

The most gratifying change occurred in the gut. It had always had a tendency to be what is termed spastic. Gas would be trapped in various segments, causing discomfort. A physician once advised dosing with a long-acting barbiturate daily to relax the intestinal musculature. I put up with the discomfort instead. The extra C erased all that, plus a hemorrhoid or two that had put in an appearance a couple of plateaus ago. Those were welcome changes. I could eat gas-generating foods and pass the proverbial peck of pine cones without a problem. One can become lyrical over such freedoms, even skip around singing that the fountain of youth bubbles up from a reservoir of pure ascorbic acid. Picture a scene of oldsters cavorting nearby, radiating the frenetic happiness of a beer commercial. High C appeared to put the aging process on hold.

Then prepare yourself for the sweet accompaniment to turn discordant, as when the villain enters. My first affliction to vanish was the first to return: the ear began to itch again. Somewhat disillusioned, I thought of dropping the high dose. A novice is fearful of taking too much because of the stories about kidney stones and such. Had I known of the iron-overload reaction with C that causes heart problems I wouldn't have started the regimen at all—not without being checked for iron status. A prudent individual would have a kidney-function test also and arrange for observation by a physician if on anticoagulants. Fortunately my kidneys were good, I wasn't on anticoagulants and iron overload is rather uncommon. The 10 weeks of heightened well being promised a better future so my initial apprehension soon faded. I raised the daily dose to 8 grams then practically set up camp in the medical library nearby to settle for myself the matter of alleged side effects ... Again, about 10 weeks later, the ear itch returned. I raised to 10 grams. Thus went the upward ratcheting of the dose about every 10 weeks, accompanied by a growing concern that the uptick might never stop. Only the extensive reading in the library kept me on course, as the findings assured me that high C is relatively harmless. Finally, at 16 grams a day, the ear itch did not return on schedule. It now bothers only occasionally when for some reason or another the body seems to need more C.

The experience teaches a great deal about the substance. Diminishing response to a given amount is definitely a factor to consider in high-C dosing, at least in the elderly. Perhaps it applies at all ages. The uselessness of small dosings with C before a cold strikes reinforces the suspicion that diminishing effectiveness—sometimes termed tachyphylaxis—can occur quickly at any age. The reaction points up the inadequacy of short-term trials on fixed doses. In order to learn more about C the trials should be continued much longer with doses that can be adjusted as needed in conformance with standard practice when treating with other drugs.

On 16 grams a day the cold sores which bothered me regularly prior to the regimen never appear. A cold may try to establish itself but cannot do so. The flu will still come on but is squelched by a rise in dose. The misery of it is avoided. There is simply no down time from these diseases anymore.

In the years since the start of high C two unexpected benefits have solidified my belief in the versatile nature of it. One involves the shrinking of a basal cell carcinoma which was growing in a typical position on my right face near the nose. The type that Reagan had. I had removed 2 others from my left face a few years before. This one was due for the same procedure at the time I began the high-C regimen but I'd kept putting it off simply because I don't relish coming at myself with an anesthetic syringe and a scalpel. A small reddish center had appeared in the dark growth, indicating that the growth was close to the scabbing stage in the spring of '86 when I started on high C. Very slowly afterward the red center disappeared and the dark body lightened to the color of a freckle and shrank, the process taking over a year. Only a small flesh-colored raised area topped with a freckle remains.

Klenner mentioned having removed this type of slow-growing skin cancer with a 30-percent C ointment (1971). For several days I tried his method on the remnant, turning it and the surrounding skin red and tender but after all had returned to normal one could see that the topical ointment had not shrunk it further. This is entirely different from the effect of C on certain types of wart. Two or three applications remove them quickly.

The second surprise came with the realization that my right eye is clear. For years I had noticed a spot as if the eyeglass on that side had a wide dash painted on it in the "4 o'clock" position. Its disappearance occurred so gradually that I can't point to the year that it vanished. This plus the skin-cancer resolution raises the thought that high C tends to work toward erasing flaws that develop during life. The slow disappearance of intestinal polyps, mentioned earlier, seems to support the idea. But high C isn't a cure-all. The "winter itch" that plagues oldsters hasn't yet been relieved by my big dose.

Not everyone is endowed with the convenient indicator of C status that my ear itch provides. A year ago a friend could not point to any benefit at all from a 10-gram daily dose as she looked back on 2 years of the regimen. She even felt it was a detriment. Never before had she endured a tickly throat and deep cough that lasted all winter. An identical experience occurred the following winter. Do we blame the 10-gram daily dose of C or say that her immune system coincidentally weakened enough to allow a persistent low-grade infection? C is a good suspect in this case. But during the last winter the tickly-cough-deep-cough condition did not occur. Again, was it coincidence or do we *credit* C this time? Because starting the previous summer she had raised her daily intake to 16 grams.

Pondering it, plus certain anecdotal accounts in other chapters, one begins to suspect that somewhere between 15 and 20 grams a daily dose range is reached that performs better than doses which are not quite up there. Perhaps an amount in the higher teens supplies a critical concentration so that C is forced past the body's processing machinery to do some good. So many instances of effective dosing are seen to fall in that range.

There are a bucketful of questions to ponder about C. For example, what are the leukocyte and plasma C levels of those spry old folks above 90 years of age? If we extend the lines which indicate the decline of C with age, those oldsters are running mighty low. But are they really? Their bodies may be more than normally efficient in the use of C. A large-scale investigation in this area would be enlightening.

But still first on the to-be-answered-scientifically list is the C-versus-colds question. Those of us who know the answer would like to ram the truth down the establishment's throat. It rankles to keep hearing the ad announcer intone, "Until there's a cure, there's ..." Whatever. We'd like a trial set up, with all the safeguards against rigging, so that individuals with starting colds would be more adequately dosed than in the past. This means flexibility—enough C supplied to keep ahead of symptoms.

Actually a cold trial was conducted which did employ an adequate dose against a placebo—8 grams a day for 4 days. It was a fixed dose but enough for many colds. C.W.M. Wilson reported it in 1975 as an incidental comment while answering a question on the possible toxicity of C. It was not a large-scale trial, however, and no mention was made of a double-blind procedure. He did not report the outcome in a direct manner. Instead, he stated that for therapeutic effect enough C must be given to maintain the leukocyte C level at normal as long as symptoms are present. It was a nice way to leave the advertisers undisturbed while hinting that C can do the job.

It would be interesting to see a medically-supervised long-term trial set up to determine whether maintaining leukocyte C levels at high normal would prevent the onset of diabetes. The general suspicion is that at least in some cases the disease commences in a predisposed individual after an inflammatory process is initiated by something in the environment, such as a virus. One thought is that a virus starts an infection, then some white cells move in to trigger a reaction in which the insulin-producing cells are destroyed by the body's own defense mechanism. The experiment would be too difficult to conduct to be practical, however. In addition to maintaining high leukocyte C levels the C intake would need to be raised promptly at the onset of every infection or other stress. It is not likely that just a high continuous intake of C starting at an early age would be preventive. There is a mention in the literature of a physician who gave his children as many grams of C a day as their age in years until at ten the dose remained at 10 grams a day from then on. The children were still subject to viral attacks. But maybe not all viruses could survive such doses.

From a practical angle, more needs to be learned

about C and anticoagulants. Those who are on such drugs have good reason to avoid more than a gram of C daily because higher doses have caused a shortening of the clotting time in some individuals, as mentioned. Yet some folks on anticoagulants probably could benefit from high-dose C. Vitamin C itself is a moderate anticoagulant (C.A. Owen, 1970). Would C in high doses multiply that effect so that anticoagulants could be eliminated altogether? Perish the thought, say the drug companies but the reason for the thought is this: a friend's clotting time used to be short. On a daily dose of C above 10 grams, however, it is long.

These are the sort of musings which cause healthcare personnel to tear their hair. It reflects the genuine concern that people can do the damnedest things when they read that taking a vitamin or mineral might be a good thing. The dose and conditions can be garbled in perception and result in overdosage with unfortunate results. Examples abound.

An account by W.P. Patterson in 1985 is a good one. A man read that zinc might help his prostate problem so he began taking 450 milligrams a day, 30 times the recommended dose. Taking that multiple of C beyond the recommended dose creates no problem but zinc is different. The man took the 450 milligrams of zinc for 2 years before he saw a doctor to complain that he'd been tired for the past 6 months and had developed angina, shortness of breath and other ailments. He was found to have severe anemia of the type due to poor production of hemoglobin. The high zinc intake had depleted the body of necessary copper and blocked any new absorption by the gut. Luckily, the man recovered about 3 months after the high zinc dose was stopped.

You'll recall in the chapter on history that a young man was found to have a high level of plasma C after taking 10 grams a day for 4 months. He took the high dose because of a leg infection and had heard that C cures infections. It did not heal, however, after 4 months of treatment. He had to see a doctor after all. The extra C did not hurt him but such actions irritate healthcare professionals who feel that a little knowledge is a dangerous thing.

The picture of a car stunting on TV is often accompanied by a caution not to try the stunt with your own car. Likewise, these musings and the medical reports cited here are accompanied by a caution that none of it is medical advice. It is a clearing up of misconceptions, a passing on of more than just a little information and a needling of the establishment to lighten up on C.

Many an authority signals a personal disgust toward the practice of ingesting large amounts of C, using words like fad, popular folly or abuse in their discussions. Comments of this sort are diminishing as the benefits of high doses for some individuals become known. But residual disdain is still with us.

The wife of a public health official in my area developed multiple sclerosis. I suggested that she might like to know that high doses of C had been helpful. He soured and turned away, not even willing to inquire about the source of my information. Two more victims of the disease are afraid to try it because they're afraid their doctors wouldn't approve. There is nothing in recent widely circulated literature which would alert physicians to the 40-year-old information on C in the treatment of multiple sclerosis. Irwin Stone's 1982 paper which called attention to the near-scurvy condition of multiple sclerosis patients appeared in a journal with limited circulation.

The abridged medical index, the publication whose purpose is to provide physicians with practical information of immediate value, did not list the article. As mentioned, it also omitted reference to the 1973 paper which reported on the disruptive blood condition when a cold strikes and the necessary preventive dose. Also passed up: Basu's paper on relief of bone pain in Paget's disease by C; Cathcart's 1984 paper on the treatment of AIDS with high C; and the 1990 paper by Harakeh on the suppression of the AIDS virus by an amount of C which is easily achieved in the plasma by oral dosing.

A recent textbook on AIDS compares in size with a stack of 5 *National Geographics*. Imagine how much information it contains! How much on vitamin C as a beneficial treatment?

Nothing.

No wonder physicians don't know what they need to know about C. A not-so-mysterious force out there doesn't want them to know.

NOTES

1. G. Schectman's investigation suggests that smokers may need a C intake of 200 milligrams or more daily to equal the nonsmoker's C status (1991).

2. The journal Medical Hypotheses does carry some advertising but hasn't attracted much interest from large drug companies.